Clinical Tropical Medicine

Clinical Tropical Medicine

G.O. Cowan
Director of Army Medicine, Ministry of Defence,
Royal Army Medical College, London

and

B.J. Heap
Consultant in Communicable Disease Control,
Norwich District Health Authority

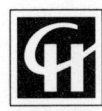

CHAPMAN & HALL
London · Glasgow · New York · Tokyo · Melbourne · Madras

Published by Chapman & Hall, 2–6 Boundary Row, London SE1 8HN

Chapman & Hall, 2–6 Boundary Row, London SE1 8HN, UK

Blackie Academic & Professional, Wester Cleddens Road, Bishopbriggs, Glasgow G64 2NZ, UK

Van Nostrand Reinhold Inc., 115 5th Avenue, New York NY10003, USA

Chapman & Hall Japan, Thomson Publishing Japan, Hirakawacho Nemoto Building, 6F, 1-7-11 Hirakawa-cho, Chiyoda-ku, Tokyo 102, Japan

Chapman & Hall Australia, Thomas Nelson Australia, 102 Dodds Street, South Melbourne, Victoria 3205, Australia

Chapman & Hall India, R. Seshadri, 32 Second Main Road, CIT East, Madras 600 035, India

First edition 1993

© 1993 Chapman & Hall

Typeset in 11/12½pt Palatino by Acorn Bookwork, Salisbury, Wiltshire
Printed in Great Britain by the University Press, Cambridge
ISBN 0 412 43330 3   0 442   (USA)

Apart from any fair dealing for the purposes of research or private study, or criticism or review, as permitted under the UK Copyright Designs and Patents Act, 1988, this publication may not be reproduced, stored, or transmitted, in any form or by any means, without the prior permission in writing of the publishers, or in the case of reprographic reproduction only in accordance with the terms of the licences issued by the Copyright Licensing Agency in the UK, or in accordance with the terms of licences issued by the appropriate Reproduction Rights Organization outside the UK. Enquiries concerning reproduction outside the terms stated here should be sent to the publishers at the London address printed on this page.
    The publisher makes no representation, express or implied, with regard to the accuracy of the information contained in this book and cannot accept any legal responsibility or liability for any errors or omissions that may be made.

A catalogue record for this book is available from the British Library

Library of Congress Cataloging-in-Publication data available

∞ Printed on permanent acid-free text paper, manufactured in accordance with the proposed ANSI/NISO Z 39.48-199X and ANSI Z 39.48-1984

Contents

Foreword   xi

Part One   Protozoal Diseases

1 Malaria   **3**
   Introduction   3
   Epidemiology and transmission   3
   Pathogenesis   5
   Clinical features   8
   Diagnosis   10
   Differential diagnosis   11
   Laboratory investigations   11
   Treatment   12
   Prevention and control   18
   Personal prophylaxis   18

2 Visceral Leishmaniasis (Kala-azar)   **23**
   Epidemiology   23
   Clinical features   26
   Diagnosis   27
   Treatment   28
   Prevention and control   29

3 Cutaneous Leishmaniasis (*David S. Jolliffe*)   **31**
   Introduction   31
   Epidemiology   31
   Pathogenesis, pathology and immunology   32
   Clinical features   34
   Diagnosis   36
   Therapy   37
   Prevention and control   38

4 African Trypanosomiasis   **39**
   Epidemiology   39

	Clinical features	42
	Diagnosis	43
	Treatment	44
	Prevention and control	45
5	**American Trypanosomiasis**	**47**
	Epidemiology	47
	Clinical features	49
	Diagnosis	51
	Treatment	52
	Prevention and control	52
6	**Amoebiasis**	**55**
	Aetiology and epidemiology	55
	Clinical features	56
	Diagnosis	60
	Treatment	63
	Prevention and control	65
7	**Giardiasis**	**67**
	Aetiology and epidemiology	67
	Clinical features	68
	Diagnosis	69
	Treatment	70
	Prevention and control	71
8	**Cryptosporidiosis**	**73**
	Aetiology and epidemiology	73
	Clinical features	73
	Diagnosis	74
	Treatment	74
	Prevention and control	74

Part Two   Helminthiases

9	**Roundworm Diseases**	**77**
	Ascariasis	77
	Hookworm Disease	80
	Strongyloidiasis	83
	Trichinosis	85
	Trichuriasis	87
	Visceral Larva Migrans	88
10	**Tapeworms (Cestodes)**	**89**
	Taenia saginata	89

	Taenia solium	91
	Hydatid disease	95
	Echinococcus granulosus	95
	Echinococcus multilocularis	98
11	**Filariasis and Onchocerciasis**	**101**
	Introduction	101
	Lymphatic filariasis	101
	Loiasis	105
	Mansonella perstans (Dipetalonema perstans)	106
	Mansonella streptocerca	106
	Onchocerciasis	106
	Dracontiasis	108
12	**Schistosmiasis and Human Fluke Infections**	**111**
	Schistosomiasis	111
	Liver fluke diseases of man	114
	Intestinal flukes in man	118
	Lung flukes or paragonimiasis	122

Part Three   Bacterial Diseases

13	**Tuberculosis**	**129**
	Introduction	129
	Epidemiology and pathogenesis	129
	Pulmonary tuberculosis	130
	Lymph node tuberculosis	134
	Tuberculosis of the pericardium	136
	Abdominal tuberculosis	138
	Genitourinary tuberculosis	141
	Tuberculosis of the spine	142
	Tuberculous meningitis	144
	Tuberculosis and human immunodeficiency virus	147
14	**Leprosy**	**149**
15	**Leptospirosis and Relapsing Fever**	**155**
	Leptospirosis	155
	Relapsing fever	158
16	**Acute Bacterial Meningitis**	**161**
	Meningococcal meningitis	161
	Haemophilus influenzae meningitis	165
	Pneumococcal meningitis	167
	Bacterial meningitis – organism not identified	167

17	**Enteric Fever**	**169**
18	**Tetanus**	**173**
19	**Sexually Transmitted Diseases**	**175**
	Genital ulcer disease	175
	Urethral discharge in males	180
	Vaginal discharge	181
	Pelvic inflammatory disease	182
	Ophthalmia neonatorum	183
20	**Brucellosis and Melioidosis**	**185**
	Brucellosis	185
	Melioidosis	186
21	**Anthrax, Tularaemia and Plague**	**187**
	Anthrax	187
	Tularaemia	188
	Plague	188
22	**Rickettsial Diseases**	**191**
	Typhus and the spotted fever group	191
	Coxiella burneti (Q fever)	199
	Human ehrlichiosis	200

Part Four Diarrhoeal Diseases

23	**Diarrhoeal Diseases**	**205**
	Acute watery diarrhoea	205
	Cholera	205
	Vibrio parahaemolyticus	209
	Non-typhoidal salmonellosis	209
	Enterotoxigenic *Escherichia coli* (ETEC)	210
	Enteropathogenic *Escherichia coli* (EPEC)	211
	Clostridium perfringens	212
	Dysentery	213
	Shigellosis	213
	Enterohaemorrhagic *Escherichia coli* (EHEC)	215
	Enteroinvasive *Escherichia coli* (EIEC)	216
	Campylobacter enteritis	216
	Yersinia enterocolitica	217
	Chronic diarrhoea	217

Part Five   Viral Diseases

24	Arboviruses	223
25	Acquired Immunodeficiency Syndrome	231
	Clinical features	232
	Human T lymphotrophic virus 1	235
26	Hepatitis	237
27	Rabies	243

Part Six   Fungal and Skin Diseases

28	Fungal Infections	249
29	Skin Ulcers	253
30	Myiasis	255

Part Seven   Nutritional Diseases and Poisoning

31	Nutritional Deficiencies and Poisoning	259
	Protein energy malnutrition	259
	Vitamin A deficiency	262
	Beri-beri	263
	Pellagra	263
	Rickets	264
	Goitre and cretinism	265
	Organophosphate poisoning	265
	Tropical ataxic neuropathy	266
	Lathyrism	266
32	Snake Bite	267

Part Eight   Eosinophilia and Unexplained Fever

33	Eosinophilia	273
	Angiostrongylus cantonensis	275
34	Pyrexia of Unknown Origin	277
	History	277
	Examination	277
	Investigation plan for fever after tropical exposure	280

x Contents

Part Nine Travelling to the Tropics

35	**Outlines of Immunization and Protection of the Traveller**	**285**
	Immunizations	285
	International travel, sexually transmitted diseases and HIV	290
	Traveller's diarrhoea	291
	Prevention of malaria	293
	Heat illness	293

Bibliography 295

Index 303

Foreword

Tropical medicine is taught at best very briefly in most medical schools in the developed world. Although increasing numbers of their students and young graduates seek clinical experience in tropical countries, those who remain at home must expect to see increasing cases of exotic diseases in tourists, migrants and business travellers.

The thriving existence of post-graduate diploma and master's courses in tropical medicine in both Europe and North America testify to such a requirement for knowledge in the field of tropical disease, which is also evidenced by the publication of several large text-books dedicated to the subject. Our own recent experience in the teaching and examining of tropical medicine courses in Britain has taught us that there is a need for a concise up-to-date paperback textbook giving a comprehensive coverage of clinical tropical medicine and is aimed at doctors on these courses, medical students on tropical electives, and physicians practising in infectious diseases and the primary and hospital care of travellers.

This book is based on considerable experience of the practice of medicine in local populations in the Far East, Nepal, India, East and West Africa and tropical Australia. In order to keep the size of the book within reasonable bounds, we have been unable to cover the very important fields of anaemia, cardiovascular, renal and neurological disease in tropical medicine. Some of the investigations and treatments we describe are not available in the tropics, but have been included to help those treating tropical diseases in developed countries.

Our special thanks are due to Mrs Matilda White for her work in typing part of the manuscript and to our colleague Colonel David Jolliffe FRCP for his Chapter on cutaneous leishmaniasis, on which he is an international expert.

The ethos of this book can be traced to Sir Thomas Browne's words in a letter to a friend in 1657:

'Besides the common swarm, there are endemial and local infirmities proper unto certain regions, which in the whole Earth make no small number; and if Asia, Africa and America should bring in their list, Pandora's Box would swell and there must be a strange Pathology.'

G.O. COWAN
B.J. HEAP

Part One
Protozoal Diseases

1
Malaria

INTRODUCTION

Malaria was believed, until the end of the 19th century, to be caused by a 'miasma' or 'bad air' arising from swamps. It was then shown by Alphonse Laveran and Ronald Ross to be caused by protozoan parasites transmitted by anopheline mosquitoes. Human malaria is caused by four species of plasmodia – *falciparum*, *vivax*, *ovale* and *malariae* – which cause 100 million cases yearly of clinical disease, with up to two million deaths, and infect the blood of 280 million people.

EPIDEMIOLOGY AND TRANSMISSION

Malaria is widely distributed in the tropical and subtropical zones, being endemic throughout South and South-east Asia, Africa, areas of the Middle East and South and Central America.

The malaria parasites are protozoa of the genus *Plasmodium*. Four parasites give rise to malaria in man – *Plasmodium vivax*, *P. ovale*, *P. malariae*, and *P. falciparum*. The parasites are transmitted from man to man by the female anopheline mosquito. In man, the vertebrate host and reservoir, parasites multiply dividing asexually, a process called schizogony. In the mosquito parasites multiply by the sexual process of sporogony.

When an infected mosquito bites man it injects thin, spindle-shaped forms of the parasite, called sporozoites, into the blood. These are cleared from the blood in less than an hour, a proportion entering hepatocytes. In the hepatocyte the sporozoite grows and by multiple division (pre-erythrocytic schizogony) of its nucleus produces a large, multinucleate schizont. As this schizont develops each nucleus forms into a new small, elongated cell called a merozoite. When mature, the liver schizonts burst and release their merozoites into the bloodstream. With *P. falciparum*, schizogony can produce up to 40 000 merozoites per schizont while *P. vivax* may produce 10 000. In *P. vivax* and *P. ovale* latent forms, or hypnozoites, may remain dormant in the liver cells and delayed cell division may lead to relapses of malaria.

Merozoites enter red blood cells and undergo further development. The merozoites feed on the red cell haemoglobin and change progressively into trophozoites. Fully grown trophozoites divide into schizonts (erythrocytic schizogony). Mature schizouts, depending on the species, contain six to 24 merozoites, which are released into the bloodstream when the red cell ruptures. These merozoites can infect new red cells and the cycle is repeated.

The pre-patent period is the interval between infection and the time when the malarial parasites are detectable in the blood but cause no symptoms. The time interval between infection and the first appearance of clinical symptoms of the disease is called the incubation period. The incubation period for *P. falicparum* is 12 days, for *P. ovale* it is 13 to 17 days, for *P. malariae* it is 28 to 30 days, and for *P. vivax* it is usually 13 to 17 days, but may be up to 9 months.

After several generations of merozoites have been produced, some, instead of developing into schizonts, undergo sexual differentiation to become male and female gametocytes. When taken up by a feeding mosquito these gametocytes undergo further development. In the stomach of the mosquito the female gametocyte forms a macrogamete and the male a microgamete. The male gamete divides and forms a number of long, slender flagella. One of these flagella enters the female macrogamete and fuses to form a zygote. The zygote changes into a mobile ookinete which penetrates the stomach wall to form an oocyst, attached to the outer stomach wall. The oocyst grows and by multiple nuclear fission produces sporozoites. These burst through the oocyst wall and invade the mosquito's body cavity with a proportion reaching the salivary glands. The next time the mosquito feeds on man it injects the sporozoites in its salivary glands into the bloodstream, and the parasitic life cycle continues in man.

The time taken for the development of the malaria parasite in the mosquito is called the extrinsic incubation period. It varies with the different parasite and mosquito species, and environmental factors, especially temperature, but is never shorter than 9 days.

Malaria may also be transmitted by transfusion of infected blood and transplacentally. Under these circumstances liver stages, and in particular hypnozoites, are not produced.

PATHOGENESIS

Malarial fever occurs at the time of rupture of red blood cells containing mature schizonts. If this process becomes synchronized, episodes of fever occur on every second day ('tertian' fever), as in *P. vivax* and *P. ovale* infections, or on every third day ('quartan' fever), as with *P. malariae*. In *P. falciparum* disease, multiplication and invasion occur so rapidly that no synchronous pattern develops and the fever persists.

Fever in malaria results from the release of endogenous cytokines (e.g. interleukin 1 (IL-1), tumour necrosis factor (TNF)) in reaction to parasite antigens, which help to protect the patient from further invasion by enhancing the immune response and inhibiting multiplication of the parasites, but which in severe infections may potentiate damage to vital organs.

In *P. vivax*, *P. ovale* and *P. malariae* infections it is rare for more than 1% of circulating red blood cells to be parasitized; the main features of the illness are paroxysms of fever, accompanied by headaches, muscle pain and nausea, and the symptoms attributable to splenomegaly, which causes discomfort under the left lower ribs and results in accelerated destruction of red blood cells and platelets. The enlarged spleen is susceptible to damage by trauma. Massive splenomegaly due to repeated malarial immunostimulation occurs in some individuals, probably on a genetic basis, and leads to hyper-reactive (tropical) splenomegaly syndrome with a potential for the development of chronic lymphatic leukaemia.

Chronic *P. malariae* infection may cause progressive immune-complex deposition in the renal glomerular membrane, leading to nephrotic syndrome, especially in children in Africa.

The pathogenesis of 'severe and complicated' malaria, which is always due to *P. falciparum*, has been intensively studied in recent years. In the 1960s the theory of **increased capillary permeability** as the cause of the pathology prevailed. Considerable evidence has since been advanced to show that **microvascular obstruction by parasitized red cells** explains many of the disease processes. It has long been known that *P. falciparum* schizonts rarely appear in peripheral blood; it is now clear that red cells containing them

6 Malaria

Table 1.1 Mechanisms of RBC–capillary adherence in malaria

1. Increased production of **thrombospondin**, an extracellular matrix glycoprotein, in the capillary wall.
2. Increased production of leukocyte *CD 36* glycoprotein.
3. Increased production of an intracellular adhesion molecule *ICAM-1*.
4. Production of **adhesin** by parasitized RBCs – evident as surface 'electron-dense knobs'.

are sequestered in deep capillary beds throughout the body, most crucially in the brain and kidneys, and importantly in bone marrow, liver and the placenta in pregnancy. Sequestration allows the malaria parasites to avoid destruction in the spleen. This results from increased adherence by parasitized red cells to capillary endothelium through a variety of interacting mechanisms (Table 1.1).

The resulting **capillary stasis** in vital organs produces metabolic arrest, without causing total vascular occlusion (as evidenced by the lack of histological infarction in involved tissues). Brain cells in particular are unable to perform aerobic glycolysis to obtain energy and so depend on inefficient anaerobic glycolysis; this results in lactic acidosis and global brain dysfunction, leading to coma and death.

Hypoglycaemia is an important complication of *P. falciparum* malaria and may result from three separate mechanisms (Table 1.2). The significance of the accompanying **hypophosphataemia** has not yet been fully studied.

Acute **renal failure** is an important contributor to the mortality of severe malaria. It is caused by four interacting mechanisms (Table 1.3).

Progressive **anaemia** results from haemolysis of parasitized red cells and hypersplenic destruction of normal red cells, and from ischaemia of the bone marrow. Auto-immune haemolysis is not

Table 1.2 Causes of hypoglycaemia in *P. falciparum* malaria

1. Increased utilization of glucose (anaerobic glycolysis) by malaria parasites.
2. Reduced liver gluconeogenesis, due to microvascular obstruction.
3. Insulin release from pancreatic islets by quinine or quinidine used in treatment.

Table 1.3 Causes of acute renal failure in *P. falciparum* malaria

1. Hypovolaemia, due to sweating, vomiting and diarrhoea.
2. Renal vasocontriction, due to kinin release.
3. Microvascular obstruction in glomeruli and tubules.
4. Malarial pigment and haemoglobin nephropathy, due to haemolysis.

usually important. Thrombocytopenia results from hypersplenism; auto-immune antibodies and intravascular coagulation are not usually important.

The question of **increased capillary permeability** in *P. falciparum* malaria has, however, remained open for the following reasons:

1. Pulmonary oedema is common and is accompanied by neutrophil and monocyte infiltration and platelet **aggregation** which may result in respiratory distress syndrome.
2. Small children have increased intracranial pressure, although this is not found in adults with cerebral malaria.

Small intestinal capillaries are also congested with parasitized red cells; this may cause diarrhoea and acute malabsorption, and may be complicated by endotoxic shock caused by endogenous enterobacteriaceae.

New knowledge of the pathogenesis of severe malaria has prompted reseach into the possibility of modifying production of adhesin, thrombospondin, IL-1 and TNF by the production of monoclonal antibodies, but these approaches are experimental and may carry risks of suppression of normal defence mechanisms.

Immunity to malaria develops after repeated non-fatal infection, and progressively reduces the severity of each illness, but does not prevent parasitaemia, so that immune adults remain infective to mosquitoes. Illness may recur, after several years of no exposure to infection, or in immune suppression (e.g. by pregnancy or splenectomy), but there is as yet no evidence that human immunodeficiency virus (HIV) infection increases the risk of illness or death from malaria.

Immunity to malaria is specific to the species and to strains within species, and is mediated by the spleen through helper T cells. Circulating antibody to sporozoites is present in African populations, but appears to be non-protective, and antibodies to gametocytes do not occur naturally in man.

Severe childhood malnutrition is relatively protective against malaria, since the malaria parasites require iron, folic acid and glucose for multiplication. Energetic feeding regimens may lead to malarial attacks as the child recovers.

The phenomenon of **balanced polymorphism** has been shown in countries with a high incidence of malaria to provide partial protection against parasitization of red cells, in that some hereditary abnormalities confer a selective advantage for survival, e.g. haemoglobin AS, B-thalassaemia trait, ovalocytosis and Duffy-negative blood group in Africans (for *P. vivax*).

CLINICAL FEATURES

During the **incubation period** of 8 to 30 days the patient remains well, with no fever or disturbance of liver function.

The first clinical manifestation is **fever**, accompanied by headache, nausea and muscle pain (especially in the back) in a classical sequence starting with cold chills and shaking, proceeding to a hot dry stage as the fever rises, and culminating in drenching sweats as the temperature falls, lasting in all about 10 hours. Such 'paroxysms' occur every 48 hours in *P. vivax* and *P. ovale* malaria, if untreated, and every 72 hours with *P. malariae*. With *P. falciparum* no such periodicity is established; the fever may persist, or occur in daily cycles.

Most patients with malaria become anaemic and slightly jaundiced, and all have an enlarged spleen, which may cause discomfort. Accompanying symptoms and signs may include a dry cough, nose bleeds, diarrhoea and labial herpes.

P. falciparum has the potential for causing serious complications and death. 'Severe and complicated malaria' is defined by the criteria as shown in Table 1.4.

Early clinical warnings of severe malaria are provided by the features listed in Table 1.5.

Patients with fully established severe *P. falciparum* malaria may be comatose (possibly with decorticate posturing), anuric, severely hypoglycaemic and hypotensive, with evidence of pulmonary oedema.

Pregnant women with *P. falciparum* malaria experience more severe clinical illness, even if they have been previously immune, with high risks of severe anaemia, abortion or stillbirth, and maternal death, especially in primiparae.

Small children are most at risk in malarial areas from the ages of 1 to 5 years, often presenting with status epilepticus or mening-

Table 1.4 Defining criteria for severe and complicated *P. falciparum* malaria

1. Unrousable coma.
2. Severe normocytic anaemia H6 < 5g/l, PCV < 15.
3. Renal failure (urinary output under 400 ml in 24 h, serum creatinine over 265 mmol/l).
4. Pulmonary oedema or respiratory distress syndrome (usually with normal pulmonary capillary wedge pressure).
5. Hypoglycaemia – blood sugar < 2.2 mmol/l.
6. Circulatory collapse: Systolic BP < 50 mmHg (child).
   < 70 mmHg (adults).
7. Spontaneous bleeding or evidence of diffuse intravascular coagulation.
8. Repeated generalized convulsions.
9. Acidosis–arterial pH < 7.25, plasma bicarbonate < 15 mmol/l.
10. Macroscopic haemoglobinuria.

Other criteria
11. Impaired consciousness.
12. Severe generalized weakness.
13. Hyperparasitaemia (over 5% of RBCs in non-immunes).
14. Clinical jaundice.
15. Hyperpyrexia – over 40 °C.

ism, and may be hypoglycaemic and severely anaemic. Diarrhoea and vomiting can be severe. Signs of increased intra-cranial pressure should be sought. Children surviving acute attacks develop partial immunity and re-infection produces less severe illness, so that adults in endemic areas have a low parasitaemia permanently and are well apart from the effects of anaemia. A febrile illness in such an adult, unless immuno-compromised or pregnant, is likely to be caused by another infection (e.g. typhoid,

Table 1.5 Early clinical indications of severe malaria

1. Drowsiness or delirium, with or without neck stiffness.
2. Epileptic fits, especially in children.
3. Paralysis of conjugate eye movements, hypertonia, extensor plantar reflexes, absent abdominal reflexes.
4. Retinal haemorrhages.
5. Oliguria (under 800 ml/24 h).
6. Severe watery diarrhoea.
7. Hypotension (SBP under 100 mmHg).

lobar pneumonia, arbovirus) even if malarial parasitaemia is present.

Recrudescence of *P. falciparum* malaria occurs in partially immune individuals on re-infection and in non-immunes who have been treated with a drug to which the strain of parasite has become resistant. **Relapse** of malarial fever may occur weeks or months later in *P. vivax* and *P. ovale* infections if the parasite hypnozoites in the liver cells have not been eradicated by appropriate medication.

P. malariae infection may relapse after many years without fever. Liver hypnozoites have not been found; the infection is thought to remain dormant in red blood cells, possibly in the spleen.

Congenital malaria is rare, except in infants of non-immune mothers, and usually presents within 2 weeks of birth.

Transfused blood and blood fractions can transmit all species of malaria, but *P. vivax* and *P. ovale* infections acquired in this way do not relapse. Rarely, malaria is transmitted between sharers of intravenous needles used for drug abuse.

DIAGNOSIS

Malaria should be suspected in any patient with fever who has been exposed to malarious mosquitoes (in tropical countries, on air journeys, or near international airports), or to blood transfusion.

The diagnosis of malaria depends on the demonstration of stained parasites in the red cells of thick and thin blood films stained by Giemsa or Leishman methods. Films should be taken at 4 hour intervals, irrespective of fever paroxysms, until up to six sets have been obtained. Low levels of parasitaemia may present difficulties in:

1. patients who have taken prophylactic drugs which are only partially effective or have been taken irregularly;
2. patients who have received treatment which is partially effective or who have been given insufficient doses;
3. patients with partial immunity.

On strong clinical suspicion of malaria, particularly *P. falciparum*, full treatment should be instituted even if blood films are negative.

Demonstration of parasitaemia can be enhanced by the addition of a fluorescent dye (e.g. benzo-thio-carboxypurine BCP) to blood which is micro-centrifuged and the Buffy coat examined.

If malarial parasites are found in blood films, the diagnosis of the species is crucial, as the treatment regimen depends on this. *P. falciparum* infections are characterized by:

1. the presence of crescent-shaped gametocytes;
2. the absence of schizonts, except in very severe cases;
3. the predominance of small ring-shaped trophozoites, especially if multiple or binucleate;
4. high parasitaemia, especially if over 5% of red cells are parasitized.

Serological confirmation of the diagnosis and the species of malaria may be useful retrospectively in patients treated before positive blood films are obtained; serological methods are also valuable in epidemiological surveys and in screening of blood donors. IFAT and ELISA methods are used; detection of IgM antibodies indicates acute infection, of IgG, old or persistent infection.

DIFFERENTIAL DIAGNOSIS

In the diagnosis of malarial fever, the most common differentials include influenza, viral hepatitis, arboviruses, leptospirosis, relapsing fever, typhoid and typhus. In cerebral malaria it is essential to differentiate meningitis, viral encephalitis, heat stroke, poisoning (e.g alcohol, organophosphorus compounds), hypoglycaemia in diabetes, eclampsia and subarachroid or pontine haemorrhage.

LABORATORY INVESTIGATIONS

Patients with malaria have normocytic normochromic anaemia and thrombocytopenia, reflecting the severity of infection. The white blood cell count is usually normal, but in severe *P. falciparum* cases neutrophil leukocytosis occurs. Liver function tests show elevation of unconjugated bilirubin, due to haemolysis, and liver cell enzymes (AST, ALT).

Essential additional investigations in *P. falciparum* cases may include:

1. blood glucose serial measurements;
2. CSF examination to exclude meningitis or encephalitis;
3. blood urea and electrolytes, serum phosphate and calcium;
4. estimation of blood clotting factors;
5. blood gas estimations, blood pH;
6. blood cultures for Gram-negative bacteria.

TREATMENT

Various stages in the life cycle of the malarial parasites show different susceptibility to antimalarial drugs. Drugs can be placed into five groups according to their actions:

1. **Primary tissue schizonticides** inhibit the growth of the pre-erythrocytic stage of the parasite in the hepatocyte and prevent the schizonts from reaching the circulation. Examples are proguanil and pyrimethamine.
2. **Secondary tissue schizonticides** act on the latent hypnozoites of *P. vivax* and *P. ovale*. Primaquine is an example of such a drug used to achieve radical cure.
3. **Blood schizonticides** act on the asexual erythrocytic stage (schizogony) of the parasites to prevent production of schizonts and merozoites. Chloroquine is an example of this group, but drugs such as pyrimethamine, proguanil, sulphonamides, sulphones and antibiotics also have blood schizonticidal effects.
4. **Gametocytocides** destroy the sexual erythrocytic forms of the parasite thereby preventing infection of the mosquito. Primaquine is an example.
5. **Sporontocides** inhibit the formation of sporozoites in infected mosquitoes and in interrupting the parasite life cycle can prevent transmission. Examples are pyrimethamine, proguanil and primaquine.

Drug resistance

Resistance of *P. falciparum* to chloroquine was recognized in Thailand in 1959 and Colombia in 1960. Since then drug resistance has spread throughout East and South-east Asia, into East Africa and then West Africa, and can be found in parts of India, Iran and Afghanistan. Spread from the initial focus of resistance in South America has been less dramatic.

There is a graded responsiveness of *P. falciparum* to chloroquine. Sensitivity is defined as clearance of asexual parasitaemia within 7 days of commencing treatment. When clearance occurs within 7 days but is followed by early, or late, recrudescence, resistance is said to be at RI level. Resistance at RII level is present when there is a marked reduction in parasitaemia with treatment, but not complete clearance; and complete resistance RIII is present when there is no reduction of parasitaemia observed on treatment.

Reversal of resistance of *P. falciparum* to chloroquine *in vitro* by a number of unrelated drugs, e.g. cyproheptadine, has been demonstrated. This potential therapeutic avenue for improving malaria chemotherapy is currently being evaluated.

Treatment of *P. vivax*, *P. ovale* and *P. malariae*

Chloroquine, a blood schizonticide, is the treatment of choice for acute attacks. Strains of *P. vivax* with a reduced susceptibility to chloroquine have been reported, but drug resistance is not yet a significant problem.

Non-immune adults may be treated with the following regimen:

Chloroquine 600 mg base orally followed six hours later by a further dose of 300 mg. On each of the following 2 days chloroquine 300 mg is given in a single dose orally. In patients from endemic areas who are 'semi-immune' one dose of 600 mg is usually sufficient treatment.

Primaquine is required for radical cure in both *P. vivax* and *P. ovale* infections because of the existence of hypnozoites. Primaquine 7.5 mg twice daily for 14 days will normally effect a radical cure. A relatively resistant 'Chesson' strain of *P. vivax* is found in areas of South-east Asia and the western Pacific and requires doses of 15 mg twice daily for 14 days.

Primaquine may give rise to acute haemolytic anaemia in patients with glucose-6-phosphate dehydrogenase (G-6-PD) deficiency. In such patients primaquine should be given under close supervision at a dose of 45 mg weekly for 8 weeks.

Treatment of *P. falciparum*

A primary infection with *P. falciparum* in a non-immune patient requires urgent treatment. An indication of the severity of disease may be gained from a parasite count, but this can be low in the presence of severe cerebral malaria. In many areas *P. falciparum* is resistant to chloroquine. If there is any doubt as to the sensitivity to chloroquine then quinine must be used as the drug of choice.

Patients with mild or moderate disease may be treated with oral quinine. For adults 600 mg (of quinine salt) every 8 hours for 7 days; and for children 10 mg/kg (of quinine salt) every 8 hours for 7 days, are appropriate regimens. Parenteral administration of quinine is however the rule for patients with severe and complicated falciparum malaria.

In severe malaria, previously untreated patients should be given an initial loading dose of quinine to provide therapeutic blood concentrations as early as possible. Intravenous quinine should not be given as a bolus but by rate-controlled infusion. One recommended regimen is:

Quinine 16.7 mg/kg (loading dose) diluted in 10 ml/kg isotonic fluid by intravenous infusion over 4 hours, followed by 8.4 mg/kg over 4 hours, 8 hourly until the patient can swallow. Quinine can then be given orally to complete 7 days treatment.

Quinine can be given intramuscularly when facilities for intravenous administration are not available. Several dose regimens have been described. In adults and children 20 mg salt/kg loading dose followed by 10 mg salt/kg 8 hourly in adults, and 10 mg salt/kg 12 hourly in children, is a suitable regimen which is well tolerated.

Quinidine may be used as an alternative to quinine. It is more active as an antimalarial drug but has greater toxicity. There is less clinical experience of its use at the high doses required to treat severe falciparum malaria.

Mefloquine, a recently developed synthetic antimalarial, is a schizonticide, effective against chloroquine-resistant *P. falciparum*, but can only be given orally, limiting its uses in severe falciparum malaria. In mild to moderate disease it can be used for treatment in the following regimens:

For adults – 20 mg/kg given as two doses 8 hours apart.
For children – 25 mg/kg as a single dose.

Resistance to mefloquine is developing rapidly in South-east Asia, and *in vitro* 'intrinsic' resistance has been found in areas where mefloquine is not generally available.

Amodiaquine, despite its chemical similarity to chloroquine, has retained some activity against chloroquine resistant *P. falciparum*. Artemisinine (Qinghaosu), an extract from the Chinese herb *Artemisia annua*, destroys young trophozoites of *P. falciparum* and leads to rapid clearance of parasitaemia. A number of parenteral preparations are being evaluated and are giving encouraging results. Recrudescence rates may be high, particularly after oral therapy. Halofantrine is another promising, recently developed, synthetic antimalarial, active against chloroquine-resistant *P. falciparum*. As yet no parenteral formulation is available. Sulphonamide-pyrimethamine combinations such as 'Fansidar' have been used in the treatment of non-severe disease, but resistance to this combination is now also widespread.

The general principles in the management of severe falciparum malaria include early diagnosis, rapid clinical assessment, early antimalarial chemotherapy using optimal doses of appropriate parenteral agents, maintenance of correct fluid, electrolyte and acid-base balance, proper nursing care, and the prevention or early detection and treatment of complications.

Management of specific problems with severe falciparum malaria

Renal failure

It is important to establish whether there is a pre-renal failure or established renal failure with tubular necrosis. A high urinary sodium suggests that acute tubular necrosis has developed. Peritoneal dialysis or haemodialysis, where available, may be required. Initial doses of antimalarial drugs do not need to be reduced, but dosage of quinine should be reduced after two days of treatment.

Pulmonary oedema

Careful attention to fluid balance, maintenance of the central venous pressure between zero and 5 cm of water, and nursing the patient propped up at 45 degrees, will help prevent the development of pulmonary oedema. Once it has developed, pulmonary oedema is resistant to treatment. Administration of a high concentration of oxygen, potent intravenous diuretics and venesection (with return of packed cells to a severely anaemic patient) are often required.

Malaria

Hypoglycaemia

Hypoglycaemia must be suspected in all cases of severe falciparum malaria and regular monitoring of blood glucose concentration is essential. Quinine-induced hypoglycaemia may develop several days into treatment at a stage when the patient has recovered consciousness. Infusion of 5% dextrose may prevent quinine-induced hypoglycaemia in children, but not in adults. Once established, hypoglycaemia should be treated with an infusion of 50% glucose. Some patients respond to glucagon. Treatment of hypoglycaemia in fluid overloaded, oliguric patients poses a dilemma. Somatostatin analogues, (e.g. octreotide) have been used successfully to inhibit quinine-induced insulin release. If the patient is receiving peritoneal dialysis, glucose can be added to the dialysis fluid.

Hypotension

Hypotension may be secondary to dehydration, blood loss, pulmonary oedema, or septicaemia, and should be treated appropriately.

Bacterial infection is commonly associated with complicated falciparum malaria and includes both spontaneous and aspiration pneumonias, Gram-negative bacteraemia presumably originating from the gastrointestinal tract, urinary tract infections secondary to catheterization, and bacteraemia introduced via infected intravenous lines. When infection is present but remains unidentified, treatment with benzyl penicillin and gentamicin is a useful first line combination of antibiotics.

Anaemia and bleeding disorders

Anaemia should be treated with fresh blood in which both clotting factors and platelets are present. Disseminated intravascular coagulation is relatively more common in non-immune patients. Transfusion of fresh blood is the best treatment.

Cerebral malaria

Convulsions, vomiting and aspiration pneumonia are common. The patient should be nursed on his/her side and convulsions treated promptly. There is currently no role for corticosteroids in the treatment of cerebral malaria. A single intramuscular injection of phenobarbitone is an effective method of prevention of convulsions.

Hyperparasitaemia

Patients with heavy parasitaemia are at increased risk of developing the severe complications of falciparum malaria, and it has been suggested that exchange transfusions may be of benefit in these circumstances. Possible advantages include a more rapid reduction in parasite load, safe correction of anaemia in volume-overloaded patients, restoration of clotting factors and platelets, and removal of putative circulating toxins and metabolites. Exchange transfusion may not however remove sequestered parasites, make the control of therapeutic drug levels difficult, and in common with all blood transfusions increase the risk of blood-borne infections, including hepatitis B and C, and infection with HIV. The role of exchange transfusion in patients with hyperparasitaemia requires further evaluation.

Treatment in children

Vomiting often occurs in children with severe malaria and antimalarials should if possible be given by intravenous infusion. There are uncertainties over the short-term toxicity of intravenous chloroquine in children with regard to hypotension and sudden death. Chloroquine and quinine may be given by intramuscular injection in children if circumstances do not permit intravenous infusion. Precise dose determination on the basis of weight is mandatory. Oral administration of the drug should replace parenteral therapy as soon as possible.

Convulsions are common in children with severe malaria and an important cause of morbidity and mortality unless adequately treated. Fever may be treated with tepid sponging and fanning along with paracetamol, which is available as a suppository.

In areas endemic for *P. falciparum*, mothers should be encouraged to treat their infants for each and every febrile illness with an antimalarial drug until 'semi-immune' status is acquired.

Treatment in pregnancy

Treatment of malaria in pregnancy deserves special attention because acquired immunity is reduced during the second half of pregnancy, falciparum malaria tends to be more severe and there is an increased risk of miscarriage, premature labour and reduction in birth weight. Chloroquine prophylaxis should be given throughout pregnancy. An attack of malaria should be treated promptly with quinine, which in doses used therapeutically does not increase the risk of abortion. Blood glucose levels must be monitored carefully. Severe anaemia can be prevented with malarial chemoprophylaxis and folic acid supplements.

PREVENTION AND CONTROL

Global control

From 1957 a global programme of malaria eradication was co-ordinated and supported by the World Health Organization. However, by the end of the 1960s it became evident that technical problems, such as the resistance of mosquito vectors to insecticides and resistance of malaria parasites to drugs, presented serious obstacles to the eradication programme. Moreover, the administrative and financial difficulties of the developing countries was such that a revised strategy of 'malaria control' was introduced in 1969.

Measures for large scale control of the disease are designed to interfere with the cycle of the parasite within its human and mosquito hosts and fall into five broad groups:

1. Prevention of mosquitoes from feeding on man.
2. Reduction of mosquito breeding by eliminating collections of water or by altering the environment.
3. Reduction of mosquito larvae, by their destruction.
4. Reduction of adult mosquitoes, by insecticides.
5. Elimination of malaria parasites in the human host.

PERSONAL PROPHYLAXIS

Anti-mosquito measures

Physical measures to reduce the risk of being bitten by a mosquito are an inherent part of malaria prophylaxis. Long-sleeved shirts and long trousers should be worn at dusk. Insect repellent such as diethyl toluamide (DEET) can be used on exposed skin, and can be used to impregnate garments. Sleeping in properly screened rooms, under intact mosquito nets impregnated with permethrin, and the use of insecticide knock-down sprays, synthetic pyrethroid vapouriser mats and burning mosquito coils are all important ways in which personal protection from mosquitoes can be achieved.

Chemoprophylaxis

Under most circumstances physical anti-mosquito measures should be accompanied by chemoprophylaxis in all non-immunes in areas of malarial transmission. Chemoprophylaxis is necessary for all visitors to and residents of the tropics who have not lived there since infancy and so have not acquired and retained a semi-immune status. Travellers must be reminded that no chemoprophylaxis is completely effective and that malaria can occur during or after chemoprophylaxis.

The following are the recommendations of the UK Malaria Reference Laboratory and the Ross Institute:

1. In areas where malaria risk is generally low chemoprophylaxis with either weekly chloroquine or daily proguanil.
2. Where malaria risk is present and chloroquine resistance known to exist then chemoprophylaxis should be with both weekly chloroquine and daily proguanil.
3. When malaria risk is high and multi-drug resistant malaria known to be present then mefloquine weekly should be considered as an alternative to chloroquine and proguanil.
4. In Papua New Guinea, the Solomon Islands and Vanuatu transmission of malaria is intense, and in Papua New Guinea multiple drug resistant malaria is a problem. A combination of weekly Maloprim (a combination of pyrimethamine and dapsone) and chloroquine is recommended. Mefloquine is an option for short-term travellers.

Chloroquine is safe in children and during pregnancy. A cumulative dose exceeding 100 g of base carries the risk of retinopathy. Pruritus is a not uncommon side-effect in dark skinned races.

Proguanil, particularly in combination with chloroquine, may give rise to troublesome oral aphthous ulceration. Alopecia has been recorded, as has megaloblastic anaemia in patients with kidney disease.

Maloprim has been associated with the occurrence of agranulocytosis, most cases being related to a dosage of two tablets per week. It is recommended that the dose does not exceed one tablet per week.

Mefloquine hydrochloride is given for prophylaxis in an adult dose of 250 mg weekly. Nausea, vomiting and abdominal discomfort, and, to a lesser extent diarrhoea, are all common adverse effects found soon after taking the drug. Dizziness, disturbance of balance, and confusion, in some case amounting to psychotic disturbance, are less common. Mefloquine has a long half-life and the risk of cumulative raised blood levels and the risk of side-effects limit its use to short-stay travellers.

Fansidar has a significant association with blood dyscrasias and Stevens-Johnson syndrome and should not be used for malaria chemoprophylaxis. Amodiaquine has been linked to cases of agranulocytosis and liver damage and likewise cannot be recommended. Doxycycline has been used for malaria chemoprophylaxis. It is poorly tolerated because of upper gastrointestinal disturbance and its use is associated with photosensitivity.

When drugs are given for malarial prophylaxis they should always be started at least one week before travel to test for any idiosyncratic reaction and to attain steady state plasma concentrations. They must also be continued for at least four weeks after leaving the malarious area.

Self-treatment for suspected malaria with Fansidar, mefloquine, or halofantrine may have a role in the prevention of severe falciparum malaria in the traveller, particularly when chemoprophylaxis is limited by side-effects or poor compliance.

Only chloroquine and proguanil should be considered as safe in pregnancy. Systematic chemoprophylaxis should be undertaken in semi-immune pregnant women in malarial areas. Pregnancy should be avoided in non-immune women in areas endemic for *P. falciparum*, and pregnant women should be advised against travel to these areas.

Children born to non-immune women in malarious areas should have chemoprophylaxis from birth. Children born to semi-immunes in endemic areas have passive immunity for the first six months of their life, after which they are at increasing risk from malaria. Mass chemoprophylaxis of children is not currently recommended. Attacks of fever should be promptly treated with anti-malarial drugs, thus allowing the development of natural immunity without the occurrence of severe disease. Studies in The Gambia have, however, demonstrated that in children treatment alone did not have any significant effect on mortality and morbidity from malaria, but when combined with chemoprophylaxis there was a reduction in overall mortality in children aged 1 to 4 years, a reduction in mortality from probable malaria and from episodes of fever associated with malaria parasitaemia. Malaria antibody levels are depressed in children who have received chemoprophylaxis, but whether this depression is associated with any loss of clinical immunity is not yet clear and is being addressed by careful monitoring of children after cessation of chemoprophylaxis at the age of 5 years.

Malaria vaccines

An effective vaccine against malaria is not yet available. Attempts are in progress to develop stage specific vaccines against the sporozoite, merozoite and gametocyte stages of *P. falciparum*. A vaccine has been developed against a circumsporozoite protein and has been successful *in vitro* in blocking the invasion of sporozoites into human hepatoma cells. Any sporozoite vaccine will have to be 100% effective within 30 minutes to prevent all sporozoites from entering hepatocytes. A gametocyte vaccine would prevent transmission and therefore protect the community rather than the individual.

2
Visceral Leishmaniasis (Kala-azar)

The causative organism of visceral leishmaniasis (kala-azar) is an intracellular protozoan parasite of the genus *Leishmania*. The infection is often a zoonosis and is transmitted by phlebotomine sandflies. Visceral leishmaniasis is characterized by a prolonged irregular fever, hepatosplenomegaly, pancytopenia and progressive emaciation, leading to death by secondary infection if left untreated.

EPIDEMIOLOGY

Visceral leishmaniasis occurs widely in areas of tropical and subtropical Asia, Africa and America. It is currently a substantial problem in Northern India, Bangladesh, Nepal, China, East Africa (Sudan and Kenya) and South America (Brazil and Venezuela). Sporadic cases and minor epidemics appear in the Middle East and in most countries bordering the Mediterranean, including the Mediterranean islands.

The parasite

The leishmanial parasite exists in two morphological forms – an amastigote and a promastigote. The amastigote is 2–5 microns in diameter, being round or oval in shape. It has a nucleus and a rod-shaped kinetoplast which stains more densely than the nucleus. The promastigote is 10–20 microns long and has a free flagellum and an anterior kinetoplast. The amastigote is the only form of the parasite found in man while the promastigote is to be found in the sandfly gut and when leishmania are cultured.

Amastigotes ingested by the sandfly in a blood meal divide initially before transforming into free-swimming promastigotes.

Visceral leishmaniasis

Table 2.1 Species causing visceral leishmaniasis in man

Species	Reservoir	Area
L. donovani	Man	India
		Nepal
		Bangladesh
		Pakistan
		Afghanistan
		Iraq
		Iran
		Arabia
		Kenya
L. infantum	Dog	Mediterranean
	Fox	China
	Jackal	Arabia
	Rodents	SW USSR
L. archibaldi	?Man	
	?Dog	Sudan
	?Rodents	
L. chagasi	Dog	
	Fox	
	Opossum	C. and S.
	Porcupine	America
	Raccoon	

Promastigotes colonize the midgut where they rapidly divide and multiply before moving forwards to the sandfly pharynx. Infection in man follows injection of promastigotes during the bite of an infected sandfly. The promastigotes gain entrance into macrophages and round up to assume the amastigote form. Within the macrophage amastigote division takes place until large numbers of parasites occupy a vacuole within the cell which bursts releasing amastigotes which re-enter macrophages to continue multiplication within the reticuloendothelial system. A number of species of leishmania cause visceral disease in man and they are differentiated by isoenzyme typing, monoclonal antibody techniques and DNA probes. The species identified as causing visceral leishmaniasis in man are listed in Table 2.1.

The vector

Phlebotomine sandflies are very small (2–5 mm in length), brownish hairy flies with slender bodies, long legs and wings held erect over the body when at rest. Before a blood meal they are small enough to pass through the mesh of normal mosquito netting. Species that bite man belong to one of two genera: *Phlebotomus* in the Old World and *Lutzomyia* in the New. Most *Phlebotomus* species inhabit semi-arid and savannah areas in the Mediterranean region, the Middle East, and the tropics and subtropics of Africa and Asia, occasionally up to 50° north over warm land masses. Important vectors for human leishmaniasis include *P. argentipes* in India and *P. martini*, found breeding in vacated eroded termite hills in Kenya. *Lutzomyia* species are found in the tropics and subtropics of Central and South America, and occur mainly in forested areas. *L. longipalpis* is the most important vector of human disease. Phlebotomine sandflies of both sexes feed on plant juices but females require one or more blood meals for maturation of each batch of eggs and feed on a variety of mammals and other vertebrates. Most species of phlebotomine sandflies are not particularly anthropophilic, which may explain why the distribution of human leishmaniasis is often patchy, occurring in some areas but not in others. Sandflies are quiescent during the day, seeking shelter in dark moist places. When the light fades they become active and bite to obtain a blood meal. They may bite in the subdued light of caves or dense forest if disturbed during the day. Sandflies are weak noiseless fliers progressing by means of short hops. Preferring still, warm conditions, windy weather inhibits their flight and, even in a light breeze, biting does not occur. Because of their short flight range (usually not more than 100 m) sandflies remain in the vicinity of their breeding sites, near to the ground and seldom rise to the level of the first floor of a dwelling, often giving rise to foci of disease associated with particular sites or buildings.

Reservoir hosts

A number of animals are infected with leishmania species known to cause disease in man and may act as reservoir of infection. Examples are given in Table 2.1. In India the reservoir of infection appears to be man only. It is generally supposed that sporadic cases in Sudan and north Kenya are of zoonotic origin but that, during epidemics, man to man transmission takes place. In South America there is evidence that sylvatic, peridomestic and domestic transmission occurs, with dogs appearing to be an important reservoir for domestic transmission.

CLINICAL FEATURES

A granulomatous swelling may occur within a few days at the site of the sandfly bite, and in some individuals a vigorous immune response at this stage prevents dissemination of the parasite. Failing this, generalized spread to, and multiplication in, macrophages in reticuloendothelial tissues leads to the onset of fever after an interval of anything from 2 weeks to several years, most often about 3 months. Visceral leishmaniasis usually develops insidiously and at first its presence may not be suspected. Early lassitude, ill health and irregular fever may be noted, but absence of prostration is characteristic, even in the presence of high fever. The gradual onset tends to delay presentation until abdominal distension, weakness and weight loss are obvious. In contrast, the disease may be of acute onset and rapid progression in the non-indigenous traveller. These patients are more likely to develop the rare complications of severe acute haemolytic anaemia, acute renal damage, and severe mucosal haemorrhage.

The physical findings are weight loss, fever, anaemia and progressive painless hepatosplenomegaly. The spleen enlarges rapidly and eventually extends into the right iliac fossa. The liver enlarges to a lesser extent and less than 10% of patients become jaundiced. Generalized lymphadenopathy may occur, a feature more commonly encountered in African disease. Fever is generally irregular but a pattern of twice-daily peaks of temperature is described. There is drying and roughening of the skin and, in dark skinned races, further darkening of the skin, digits and umbilicus is a characteristic feature from which the disease gets its name kala-azar (black fever). Cough is a frequent symptom and epistaxis may occur. Alopecia secondary to chronic illness is notable especially in children. Invasion of jejunal and ileal enterocytes causes diarrhoea and malnutrition. Bone marrow invasion and suppression, compounded by hypersplenism, leads to progressive peripheral blood pancytopenia. Anaemia causes weakness and ankle oedema, leukopenia increases susceptibility to intercurrent infection, and thrombocytopenia produces purpuric rashes, bruising and bleeding from the nose and gums. Death is due to intercurrent infection, especially pneumonia, dysentery and tuberculosis. Patients infected with human immunodeficiency virus may suffer from accelerated visceral leishmaniasis.

Following appropriate treatment, some patients, especially those in India, develop widespread skin infection with viable leishmanial parasites; a condition known as post-kala-azar dermal leishmaniasis (PKDL), which is disfiguring and uncomfortable and also acts as a reservoir of the disease. PKDL appears to be associated with a breakdown of immune mechanisms whereby organisms take refuge in the macrophages of the skin where they are relatively inaccessible to chemotherapy.

Differential Diagnosis

The most important diagnostic distinction to be made is from lymphomas, chronic myeloid leukaemia and myelofibrosis. Other causes of marked splenomegaly to be considered include tropical (malarial) splenogemaly syndrome, brucellosis, schistosomiasis (*mansoni*) with portal hypertension, other causes of hepatic cirrhosis (e.g. alcohol) and haemoglobinopathies (e.g. thalassaemia, pyruvate kinase deficiency). PKDL must be distinguished from lepromatous leprosy.

DIAGNOSIS

Clinical diagnosis is confirmed by finding leishmania parasites on microscopic examination of tissue or blood. Splenic tissue obtained by needle aspiration is the most likely to demonstrate parasites (90% of active cases). Contraindications to splenic aspiration are a small soft spleen, children under the age of 5 years and an abnormal prothrombin, clotting or bleeding time. Marrow obtained by sternal or iliac crest puncture is the safer method and is positive in 80% of active cases. Liver biopsy and lymph node aspirations are alternative methods. Demonstration of leishmania in the peripheral blood is difficult. Prolonged examination of the buffy coat may show amastigotes in leukocytes, particularly in the Indian form of visceral leishmaniasis. Blood or aspirates can be cultured for leishmania on Nicolle-Novy-McNeal or Schneider's insect culture medium, or blood may be inoculated intraperitoneally into hamsters.

Despite the absence of an effective immune response in active visceral leishmaniasis, antibodies may be detected by a variety of techniques. The IFAT is generally considered the most satisfactory, but recently an ELISA and counter-current immunoelectrophoresis have proved useful.

The formol-gel test demonstrates the often massive elevation of gammaglobulins found in visceral leishmaniasis, but is non-specific, and may be positive in other conditions including malaria, tropical splenomegaly and African trypanosomiasis. Raised immunoglobulin levels may persist for many years after apparent cure.

The leishmanin skin test (Montenegro test) prepared from killed and phenol preserved promastigotes measures delayed hypersensitivity. It is negative in active visceral leishmaniasis and becomes positive following successful treatment only after several months.

TREATMENT

Pentavalent antimonials remain the cornerstone of specific chemotherapy. The most commonly used preparation is sodium stibogluconate (Pentostam). Sodium stibogluconate is best administered intravenously and is almost totally excreted in the urine within 24 hours. The standard dose of Pentostam for adults is 10 mg/kg given daily for 10 to 30 days depending on the local sensitivity of the parasite. Children require a relatively high dose of 15–20 mg/kg. Experimental evidence has demonstrated enhanced parasiticidal activity of antimony in a liposome drug delivery system but these observations have not yet been translated into clinical practice.

Antimony derivatives are potentially cardiotoxic and ECG T-wave flattening or inversion may develop and persist for several months. Other more transient changes, including bradycardia and arrhythmias, are infrequent, but collapse and sudden death are not unknown. It is important that intravenous Pentostam is given slowly, and its administration stopped immediately should coughing, vomiting or retrosternal pain develop.

Refractory and relapsing cases, and patients who develop PKDL, may be treated with further courses of sodium stibogluconate. Pentamidine and amphotericin B have been advocated as second-line drugs but both have considerable toxicity. Drugs currently under evaluation for the treatment of visceral leishmaniasis include allopurinol ribonucleoside, aminosidine (paromomycin), eflornithine, sodium aurothiomalate and interferon gamma. There is no satisfactory test of cure and patients must be followed up clinically to detect relapse. Recourse to splenectomy may be necessary when the disease is resistant to all forms of chemotherapy. Splenectomy removes the main reservoir of infection and corrects hypersplenism, and should be followed by a further course of chemotherapy. Splenectomy is attended by a subsequently increased risk of malaria and pneumococcal infections.

PREVENTION AND CONTROL

There is no effective form of immunoprophylaxis or chemoprophylaxis against visceral leishmaniasis.

Vector control

Depending upon the habits of the local vector attempts can be made to remove sandfly breeding sites. Walls of houses can be plastered and piles of rubble near dwellings removed. If termite mounds or animal burrows are breeding sites, they can be destroyed.

Sleeping areas should if possible be raised above ground-floor level. Although sandflies can pass through the mesh of mosquito nets, impregnation of nets with an insecticide such as permethrin will prevent their passage. Repellents on the skin can be used for temporary personal protection.

Spraying of houses with residual insecticide will rid homes of sandflies in areas where they are endophagic. Residual insecticide spraying against mosquitoes in malarial control programmes reduced the incidence of visceral leishmaniasis. The cessation of DDT spraying for malaria control in India, Bangladesh and southern Iran has been followed by major epidemics of visceral leishmaniasis.

Reservoir elimination

Where the domestic dog is known to act as a reservoir of infection then active case finding of sick dogs and their destruction has proven to be an effective control measure. Where man is the main reservoir then active case finding, especially of PKDL, and treatment is required. In areas where the disease is a rodent zoonosis and infection sporadic then control of the reservoir is difficult.

Manipulation of man's behaviour

Wherever possible man should avoid dwelling close to vector breeding sites or the habitat of known animal reservoirs. Large numbers of Leishmanin negative people should not be moved into an endemic area or an epidemic is likely to ensue.

3
Cutaneous Leishmaniasis

David S. Jolliffe

INTRODUCTION

Cutaneous leishmaniasis (CL) is a specific infectious granuloma transmitted by sandflies and caused by invasion of the dermis by protozoal parasites of the genus *Leishmania* which are widely distributed throughout Africa, Asia and countries bordering the Mediterranean basin (Old World) and Central and South America (New World). Although the clinical form produced by such invasion is governed by many factors, the species of the infecting parasite is of prime importance in determining the morphology of the resultant pathology which ranges from a localized self-healing lesion to a more widespread, persistent and potentially destructive disease process.

EPIDEMIOLOGY

The genus *Leishmania* consists of numerous, morphologically similar, parasites which are well adapted to survive in a wide range of mammalian and other vertebrate hosts. The species of dermatological concern in the Old World are *L. tropica*, *L. major*, *L. donovani infantum* and *L. aethiopica* whilst those from the New World are of the *L. mexicana* and *L. braziliensis* complexes. The parasitic life cycle depends on passage through the gut of a phlebotomine sandfly where the oral or rounded, intracellular, aflagellate amastigotes develop an anterior flagellum to become motile, infective promastigotes which multiply by binary fission. They migrate to the pharynx and are subsequently introduced into the host by regurgitation during the blood meal of an infected female sandfly. Within the host dermis, the promastigotes once again become amastigotes after invasion of local monocytes and loss of their flagella.

The sandfly vectors (*Phlebotomus* spp. of Old World and *Lutzomyia* spp. of New World disease) are weak, noiseless flyers with a short life-span and short flight range whose habitat is determined by the suitability of available breeding sites. Most phlebotomus species inhabit the subtropics of Africa and Asia and the semi-arid and savannah areas of the Mediterranean basin and Middle East, whilst the *Lutzomyia* species are found in forested areas in the tropics and subtropics of Central and South America. Both sexes feed on plant juices but females also require one or more blood meals for the maturation of their eggs. They are not particularly anthropophilic which probably explains why human leishmaniasis infection tends to be sporadic and confined to discrete geographical areas. The sandflies are essentially night fliers and feeders, preferring the safety of dark, moist areas during daylight hours. They are small enough to pass through the mesh of normal mosquito netting before a blood meal but their short mouthparts make them unsuited for feeding through clothing.

The cutaneous leishmaniases of man are zoonoses. In most foci of Old World cutaneous disease the reservoirs are dogs, rodents (gerbils, hyraxes and sand rats, etc.) and other small vertebrates. A greater diversity of reservoir hosts is found in the New World where sloths, armadillos, anteaters, opossums and several species of rodent have been identified. Dogs play very little part in the spread of leishmaniasis in the New World and have only been implicated in Peru where they act as reservoir for one specific form of localized disease (Uta).

Although some workers believe that man himself is the reservoir for some species of *Leishmania* causing cutaneous disease, there is little evidence to support this view.

PATHOGENESIS, PATHOLOGY AND IMMUNOLOGY

CL, like its visceral form and leprosy, is a spectrum of disease with clinical and histological patterns dependent on the cell mediated immune (CMI) response of the host. CL is, however, rather more complicated than leprosy in this regard, as clinicopathological responses are also dependent on the species of infecting leishmania.

In the centre of this spectrum, where CMI is unimpaired, the skin lesions tend to be single or few and self healing. In these forms (Oriental sore [*L. tropica*] and Chiclero's ulcer [*L. mexicana*

mexicana]), the invading promastigotes are engulfed by dermal macrophages to become infecting, intracellular, aflagellate amastigotes. They multiply by binary fission and infect adjacent macrophages which accumulate at the site of inoculation. This focus of infection soon becomes isolated and surrounded by a protective lymphocytic/epithelioid cell infiltration. Inflammation and tissue necrosis results and a spreading but usually painless ulcer is formed. Granuloma formation follows with eventual resultant healing and the formation of a characteristic scar.

At one extreme of the spectrum there is, as in lepromatous leprosy, a specific absence of CMI to the infecting leishmania. A chronic, non-ulcerative lesion develops at the site of inoculation. Leishmania are found free or in parasite laden macrophages and lymphocytic elements are conspicuous by their absence. Leishmania are disseminated widely throughout the skin and the result is the widespread, symmetrical development of nodular dermal lesions most commonly seen on the limbs and face. This anergic state is the so-called DCL caused by *L. aethiopica*, *L. m. amazonensis* and *L. m. pifanoi*.

At the other spectral pole there is an allergic, tuberculoid or lupoid form, characterized histologically by an absence of amastigotes, a heavy lymphocytic infiltration, giant cells and a few epithelioid cells. This hypersensitive state is the so-called leishmaniasis recidiva. A similar, but belated, exaggerated immune response is responsible for the development of mucocutaneous leishmaniasis (*L. braziliensis braziliensis*). In such cases, the leishmania migrate to remote dermal and mucous membrane sites before the onset of the allergic response which promotes the development of a necrotizing granulomatous reaction with the formation of micro-abscesses and an intense inflammatory cellular infiltrate leading to gross destruction of host tissues.

The development of CMI in response to infection is accompanied by delayed hypersensitivity which can be measured by the Montenegro or Leishmanin skin test. Except in DCL, a positive induration in response to the intradermal injection of killed and phenol preserved leishmanial promastigotes develops during the active stage of infection in all forms of cutaneous disease, and remains so after natural or therapeutically aided recovery. As with the Lepromin test, a proportion of the population within an endemic area will also give positive responses without showing evidence of clinical disease. This almost certainly reflects previous exposure to leishmanial organisms as the percentage of such

Leishmanin positive individuals increases with age to over 90% in some endemic areas.

Infection with all forms of cutaneous disease which is allowed to resolve spontaneously will confer immunity against reinfection with the homologous strain. Such immunity lasts for years, often for life, but reinfection with *L. tropica* has been described after many years and usually after immunosuppressive therapy. There is some cross-immunity between leishmanial strains but this is by no means always reciprocal. *L. tropica* protects against *L. major* and *L. braziliensis* protects against *L. mexicana* but in neither case is the reverse true.

CLINICAL FEATURES

Although there is considerable overlap in clinical appearance of the various forms of CL, they can usefully be described under the separate headings of localized, mucocutaneous and other forms of cutaneous leishmaniasis (Table 3.1).

Localized cutaneous leishmaniasis

This is the most common form of the disease and, as with other protozoal infections, the incubation period is variable, depending on the virulence and size of the infecting dose. After a few weeks, one or more painless itchy papules with surrounding inflammation and induration appear on exposed areas of skin. Lesions increase in size to form nodules 1 cm or more in diameter which become surmounted by an adherent crust which, on separation, reveals a shallow ulcer with a granulomatous base and an indurated, overhanging edge. The majority of untreated ulcers have healed completely within 9 months and few survive more than a year.

Variations from the above clinical picture are frequent and depend on the nature of the infecting parasite and the state of health of the patient. Each parasite produces its own spectrum of disease with considerable clinical overlap.

Acute nodular necrosis of *L. major* is typical of the 'wet', rural form which is characterized by severe ulceration with prominent serous oozing, much surrounding inflammation and lymphadenitis (Baghdad boil) whilst the more chronic 'dry' urban lesions of *L. tropica* are less dramatic and slower to heal (Oriental sore). The destruction of pinna cartilage characteristic of textbook Chiclero's

Table 3.1 Cutaneous leishmaniasis

Old World cutaneous leishmaniasis

Cutaneous	L.(tropica) major	Baghdad boil (Rural 'wet')
	L.tropica (minor)	Oriental sore (Urban 'dry')
	L.donovani infantum	
Diffuse cutaneous	L.aethiopica	
Recidiva	L.tropica	
Mucocutaneous	(L.aethiopica)	
Post kala-azar	L.donovani	

New World cutaneous leishmaniasis

Cutaneous	L.mexicana mexicana	Chiclero's ulcer
	L.m.amazonensis	
	L.m.pifanoi	
	L.braziliensis braziliensis	
	L.b.panamensis	Pein bois
	L.b.guyanensis	
	L.b.peruviana	Uta
Diffuse cutaneous	L.m.amazonensis	
	L.m.pifanoi	
Mucocutaneous	L.b.braziliensis	Espundia

ulcer caused by *L. m. mexicana* is more a reflection of the difficulty forest workers have in protecting their ears from insect bites than any particular affinity of the parasite for this particular anatomical site.

Mucocutaneous leishmaniasis (espundia)

Classically caused by *L. b. braziliensis* infection, similar lesions also develop when *L. aethiopica* infection is sited at mucocutaneous junctions. The initial lesions are indistinguishable from localized disease, but months or years later metastatic lesions appear as fungating ulcers involving the mucocutaneous junctions, particularly the nose, mouth, pharynx and larynx. Chronic progression leads to cartilage destruction, gross disfigurement and often death due to secondary infection, pneumonia or cachexia.

It is impossible to predict whether infection with *L. b. braziliensis* will progress to espundia. The reported incidence of mucocutaneous metastasis varies from 2% in Panama to 80% in Paraguay but, as in many endemic countries, documentation is poor. The metastatic disease does not resolve spontaneously and vigorous treatment with the best available therapy is therefore mandatory for all infections caused by L. braziliensis.

Other forms of cutaneous leishmaniasis

Leishmaniasis recidiva (lupoid)
An uncommon Old World syndrome caused by infection with L. tropica which differs from simple Oriental sore in that, after the primary lesions have healed, new satellite lesions virtually indistinguishable from lupus vulgaris continue to develop around the scar. It is difficult to treat and facial lesions may spread relentlessly with eventual involvement of mucous membranes.

Diffuse cutaneous leishmaniasis
Caused by infection with L. aethiopica, L. m. amazonensis and L. m. pifanoi, this form of disease is characterized by the widespread and symmetrical development of non-ulcerating nodules, most often on the face and the extensor aspects of the limbs. As in lepromatous leprosy (with which it can be clinically confused), patients mount no cellular immune response to the infecting organisms which can be readily isolated from the skin. As in the mucocutaneous and recidiva forms, treatment is very difficult.

DIAGNOSIS

As in every other field of medicine, it is of paramount importance to take a good clinical history which must include the vital question, 'Where have you travelled and when?', to determine if the patient has visited an endemic area.

Differential diagnosis includes other chronic painless ulcerating or non-ulcerating lesions such as tuberculosis, atypical mycobacterial infections, sarcoidosis, syphilis, sporotrichosis or epitheliomata. Lepromatous leprosy closely resembles the disseminated form and nasopharyngeal disease must be distinguished from blastomycosis and rhinoscleroma.

Definitive diagnosis requires the demonstration of leishmania which can be obtained most effectively from beneath the edge of the ulcer by use of a dental broach or by impression smears from the cut surface of a biopsy taken from the ulcer edge. Direct staining and examination of smears and sections so made might reveal the intracellular amastigotes (so called Leishman-Donovan or LD bodies) but more success is likely to be provided by culture of teased or biopsy material.

In old lesions, particularly those of mucocutaneous disease, parasites are usually very scanty. Useful confirmatory evidence can be obtained by a positive Montenegro test but high levels of false positive results can restrict its usefulness. A negative result in the presence of a positive parasitological diagnosis confirms DCL. Immunofluorescent antibody (IFA) tests and enzyme-linked immunosorbent assay (ELISA) techniques are becoming more and more useful as diagnostic tools with the development of specific leishmanial antigens.

THERAPY

Current treatment available for the cutaneous forms of leishmaniasis, which include chemo-, antibiotic, physical and surgical therapy, is still far from satisfactory and is the subject of ongoing, progressive clinical research.

Localized cutaneous leishmaniasis known not to be caused by *L. braziliensis* may be left to heal spontaneously or treated by curettage, local application of heat, infiltration with pentavalent antimonials or topical applications of paromomycin. If infection with *L. braziliensis* is proven or strongly suspected it must be treated to prevent mucocutaneous disease and the treatment of first choice is still with one or more courses of pentavalent antimony (Pentostam or Glucantime) in a single daily intravenous dose of 10–20 mg Sb/kg body weight with a maximum daily dose of 850 mg Sb for 20 days. Although these drugs are potentially toxic and contraindicated in patients with significant cardiac, renal or liver disease, they are generally safe and well tolerated.

Established espundia not responding to antimonial therapy may do so with amphotericin B or the aromatic diamidine, pentamidine. Both these drugs are extremely toxic but both have a place to play, alongside the pentavalent antimonials, in the treatment of DCL.

PREVENTION AND CONTROL

Transmission of New World disease occurs sporadically in a vast area of primary and secondary forest where the use of insecticide to control the sandfly population would be both ineffective and undesirable. Control of sloths and anteaters close to settlements may be of limited help but the mainstay of prevention rests with education and personal protection. Avoidance of movement in forested areas after nightfall and the use of sensible clothing, insect repellents and small mesh mosquito netting are all important. Rodent and dog control is helping to reduce the incidence of Old World disease but it is no substitute for personal protection.

Vaccination using live *L. major* has long been practised to control Old World disease. This practice has been further developed in Israel and the USSR and involves the inoculation of *L. major* promastigotes into an area of cosmetically acceptable skin. Immunity takes 2–3 months to develop and the not infrequent development of large unsightly ulcers (and subsequent scars) makes this an unsatisfactory procedure. Such vaccination is potentially extremely dangerous in the New World as only *L. braziliensis* infection will confer universal immunity. Promastigotes of *L. braziliensis* that can be guaranteed not to have the capacity to induce espundia have not so far been isolated.

Long-term chemoprophylaxis is not feasible for residents of an endemic area but the development of a suitable orally administered drug would have potential use for occasional visitors.

4

African Trypanosomiasis

African trypanosomiasis or sleeping sickness is caused by species of the *Trypanosoma brucei* group of flagellated protozoan parasites. It is transmitted to man by the bite of an infected tsetse fly of the genus *Glossina*, the distribution of which confines the disease to areas of sub-Saharan Africa. There are two species, *T. b. gambiense* and *T. b. rhodesiense*, known to cause disease in man. *T. b. gambiense* gives rise to a slowly progressive meningoencephalitis ('sleeping sickness') leading to dementia and death. *T. b. rhodesiense* causes a more acute and virulent disease which is often rapidly fatal. Recent estimates indicate that some 45 million people live in endemic areas. Of these only 5 million are under regular surveillance and 10 000 cases of human trypanosomiasis are recorded annually in Africa. The incidence of human trypanosomiasis has risen steeply in recent years because of political turmoil and population movements between infected and uninfected areas. There is no evidence as yet of increased susceptibility to trypanosomiasis in HIV infected individuals.

EPIDEMIOLOGY

The parasite

Man is infected by inoculation of metacyclic trypomastigotes during the bite of an infected tsetse fly. The metacyclic form, which is about 15 microns long and has no flagellum, transforms into a longer and more slender trypomastigote, and multiplies extracellularly by binary fission. Parasites divide and proliferate in the skin at the site of the bite before dispersing throughout the body via the lymphatic system and by haematogenous spread. Multiplication of parasites continues both in the bloodstream and in interstitial fluid. Trypomastigotes are pleomorphic, with long slender (gracile) and short sturdy (stumpy) forms with lengths of 28 and 20 microns respectively. The slender forms possess a free flagellum and a well developed longitudinal undulating membrane. These undergo binary fission during the rising phase of the first parasitaemia and when this peaks, shorter forms appear. During the falling phase non-dividing stumpy forms become predominant. A strong immunological response is mounted against the profilerating trypomastigotes with production of antibody specific to the antigenic type predominant at the peak of parasitaemia. The immune response is targeted against a surface glycoprotein, the main antigenic component of the parasite. A number of parasites are able to survive by producing an antigenically different surface glycoprotein, a phenomenon known as antigenic variation, not by genetic mutation, but as a consequence of controlled expression of a family of antigen determining genes. The peaks and troughs of parasitaemia in the host are therefore the result of proliferation of trypanosomes with a new and different antigenic type followed by destruction of the (new) major antigenic type by the host's immune response.

Glossina species become infected with *T. brucei* when circulating slender trypomastigotes are ingested during a blood meal. In the mid and hind gut of the tsetse fly the trypomastigotes multiply by longitudinal fission before gaining access to the space between the peritrophic membrane and the gut wall, penetrating the wall of the proventriculus and reaching the salivary glands where they develop into infective metacyclic trypomastigotes. Development of parasites within the tsetse fly takes between 2 and 5 weeks. Once infected the tsetse fly remains infected for life.

The less virulent *T. b. gambiense* and the morphologically indistinguishable more virulent *T. b. rhodesiense* probably represent extremes of behaviour in man of a spectrum of similar parasites. Until such a time as these are identified and classified according to their genetic and biochemical characteristics it is still appropriate to consider *T. b. gambiense* and *T. b. rhodesiense* as distinct organisms giving rise to two classical forms of disease.

The vector

Tsetse flies belong to the genus *Glossina*, about 20 species of which are known to transmit African trypanosomiasis to man. They vary in length from 0.5 to 1.5 cm and are of a brownish-grey hue occasionally with darker bands on the abdomen. They rest with their wings overlapping scissor-like above their abdomen. A distinctive feature of the genus *Glossina* is the presence of a so-called 'hatchet cell', resembling a cleaver used by butchers, in the wing venation.

Both male and female tsetse flies feed exclusively on blood from a large variety of wild and domestic animals and from man. No species of *Glossina* feeds exclusively on one host but most show host preference. The tsetse feeds during daylight hours approximately every 2 to 3 days. A tsetse fly infected with trypanosomiasis appears to take smaller, more frequent meals, often with different hosts in the same vicinity, so facilitating the transmission of the disease.

Tsetse flies are distributed widely throughout much of tropical Africa, from the southern Sahara to the northern regions of Angola, Zambia and Mozambique. Gambian sleeping sickness occurs in endemic foci over wide areas in West and Central Africa and is transmitted by riverine tsetse flies, especially *G. palpalis* and *G. tachinoides*. These flies live and breed in vegetation close to rivers and streams and may feed on man when he makes use of the rivers for washing and his water supply. The vectors of Rhodesian sleeping sickness include *G. morsitans*, *G. pallidipes* and *G. swynnertoni*, which are less dependent on moisture and live in the drier open savannah. Those at risk from contact with these species are hunters, herdsmen and tourists whose activities take them into the bush.

Transmission of African trypanosomiasis transplacentally or by blood transfusion, although uncommon, has been documented. Other biting flies such as tabanids may be responsible for some transmission, accounting for disease acquired in areas where there are no tsetse flies.

Reservoir hosts

Gambian trypanosomiasis is spread predominantly from man to man. Occasionally a human case occurs in isolation suggesting that infection has been derived from an animal source and *T. b. gambiense* has indeed been isolated from a variety of domestic and game animals in W. Africa. Rhodesian trypanosomiasis is a disease of animals with only sporadic transmission to man. The principal reservoirs are antelope such as the bushbuck and hartebeest. Rarely man-to-man transmission takes place and can lead to epidemics as have occurred in Uganda and Kenya where *G. fuscipes*, living in a peridomestic habitat, has been identified as the vector.

CLINICAL FEATURES

Multiplication of trypanosomes at the site of the tsetse bite produces an inflammatory reaction evident as a 'chancre', a small, uncomfortable, palpable, subcutaneous nodule which increases in size over a few days to produce a visible swelling. It is associated with local lymphadenopathy and persists for 2 to 3 weeks. Trypanosomes then enter and multiply in the bloodstream to cause a remittent fever starting 10 to 20 days after the bite. In pale-skinned individuals transient non-itching circles of skin redness may be seen, and in many patients flitting areas of skin oedema occur.

In rhodesiense infection the disease may progress rapidly to produce pleural effusion, splenomegaly, anaemia, hepatitis, tibial periostitis, iridocyclitis, myocarditis and, in heavy infection, death from acute meningoencephalitis.

In gambiense trypanosomiasis the early illness is usually trivial, but chronic low-grade fever, lymphadenopathy and splenomegaly persist. Enlargement of glands in the posterior triangle of the neck is known as Winterbottom's sign which, with supraclavicular lymphadenopathy, is characteristic of gambiense trypanosomiasis.

Central nervous system (CNS) manifestations in gambiense disease commonly develop after 6 to 12 months, and usually predominate in the later stages. The first indications of CNS disease are lassitude and apathy, changes in character, personality or behaviour and the complaint of persistent headache. An inconstant finding is Kerandel's sign, in which deep pressure elicits delayed hyperaesthesia. The patient grows irritable, melancholic, emotional and depressed as memory fades, intelligence degenerates and character disintegrates. Somnolence increases during the day, but at night there may be insomnia and restlessness. Sleep inversion later gives way to periods of prolonged sleep. Fine tremors and muscular rigidity of the face, tongue and fingers become evident causing slow slurred speech and dribbling of saliva. Involuntary movements and incoordination resembling Parkinsonism develop and are associated with nodding of the head and a slow, unsteady, swaying and shuffling gait. Choreiform movements appear as a particular feature of childhood disease. The face becomes puffy, especially around the eyelids, and the lips swollen, producing the effect of dull, surly indifference, and likened to 'silent grief'. Finally global brain dysfunction and death, often from pneumonia and malnutrition, supervene after months of distressing illness.

Differential diagnosis

The chancre should be distinguished from cutaneous anthrax and the eschar of tick typhus. The toxaemic illness may be confused with malaria, visceral leishmaniasis, brucellosis, miliary tuberculosis or lymphoma. The later stages may resemble AIDS, neurosyphilis, or cerebral tuberculosis, abscess or tumour.

DIAGNOSIS

The definitive diagnosis of African trypanosomiasis depends upon detection of the parasite in blood, lymph nodes or cerebrospinal fluid (CSF). In very early cases it may also be possible to demonstrate trypanosomes by aspiration of a chancre. Towards the end of the incubation period of *T. b. rhodesiense* infection, trypomastigotes can usually be found in the blood. They may be identified in a wet unstained film when they can be seen actively moving amongst erythrocytes. Formal identification requires Romanowsky staining of a dried thick blood film. Because of fluctuations in the density of parasitaemia several daily examinations of the blood may be necessary.

A more sensitive means of detection of parasites is the technique of microhaematocrit centrifugation followed by buffy-coat examination under dark ground illumination, or the use of a miniature anion-exchange centrifugation technique (MAECT). These methods are particularly useful in the diagnosis of *T. b. gambiense* where blood parasites are less easily found. Aspiration of tissue fluid from enlarged soft lymph glands is a valuable method of demonstrating parasites in gambiense disease but is less productive in the rhodesiense form where lymphadenopathy is less common.

When the CNS is involved, trypomastigotes or similar more rounded parasitic forms may be demonstrated in the centrifuged deposit of the CSF. Suggestive evidence of CNS involvement is provided by a white cell count of over $5/mm^3$ or a protein of greater than 25 mg%, which in endemic areas are generally considered as indicative of disease. The microhaematocrit centrifugation technique applied to CSF has however demonstrated the presence of trypomastigotes in the absence of the expected elevation of leukocytes and protein levels, casting doubt on these criteria.

Serological diagnostic techniques are useful adjuncts to diagnosis particularly in disease surveillance studies. The IFAT is most commonly utilized but like other immunological tests for human trypanosomiasis can give a false positive result when there has been repeated exposure to animal trypanosomes non-pathogenic to man. The IFAT requires laboratory facilities and a positive result necessitates a return visit to the patient for detailed parasitological examination, by which time the patient may not be found. A Card Agglutination Test for Trypanosomiasis (CATT) is being developed as a simple and rapid screening test for use in the field.

TREATMENT

Treatment is dependent on the use of suramin and pentamidine for early cases and melarsoprol for late stages with CNS involvement.

Suramin is the treatment most widely recommended for early sleeping sickness. A test dose of 100 mg intravenously is given in case of anaphylaxis; thereafter 20 mg/kg is given intravenously on days 1, 3, 7, 14 and 21. Suramin is nephrotoxic and the urine should be tested for protein before each injection is given. If significant proteinuria or a raised blood urea is found then treatment with suramin must stop and an alternative treatment given. Pentamidine in a dose of 4 mg/kg daily intramuscularly for 10 days can be used to treat early gambiense, but not rhodesiense, sleeping sickness. Profound hypotension can occur if pentamidine is given intravenously. Melarsoprol is also effective in the treatment of early sleeping sickness. A dose of 2.5 ml of a 3.6% solution is given intravenously on days 1 and 3 followed by 5 ml on each of days 5 and 8. Adverse reactions are rarely encountered when melarsoprol is used in this regimen.

Suramin is not effective in late disease with involvement of the CNS, as it penetrates poorly into the CSF, so treatment with melarsoprol is required. One or two injections of suramin are given first to prevent the severe febrile reaction sometimes seen when patients have their first dose of melarsoprol. Melarsoprol, a trivalent arsenical compound in 3.6% solution, is given in the dose 0.1 ml/kg (maximum 5 ml) intravenously for 4 days, and repeated three or four times after 7 day intervals in more severe cases. Melarsoprol itself can cause encephalopathy in approximately 5% of patients and this may respond to treatment with dimercaprol. Steroids are also given on empirical grounds in the belief that the melarsoprol-induced encephalopathy is partly due to an immune response rather than the toxicity of the drug. In some 5% of patients relapses occur after treatment with melarsoprol. When this occurs subsequent courses of melarsoprol should be given in combination with nitrofurazone.

Recent promise has been shown by oral eflornithine (DFMO) 400 mg/kg daily for 6 weeks in gambiense disease resistant to melarsoprol, or where the arsenical agent has proved too toxic. Patients treated for rhodesiense disease should be followed for 2 years, and those with gambiense disease for three. A lumbar puncture should be performed every 6 months to look for evidence of relapse. An increasing number of cells or elevation of protein in CSF or the persistence of a raised CSF IgM for longer than one year after treatment suggests reactivation of the disease.

Successfully treated sleeping sickness does not confer any protective immunity to reinfection.

PREVENTION AND CONTROL

There is no effective form of immunoprophylaxis and chemoprophylaxis is rarely practical. Six-monthly injections of pentamidine have been used to prevent infection in high risk groups. However, uncertainty about duration of effectiveness, reports of drug resistance, and the possibility that an existing infection may be suppressed, without cure, permitting invasion of the CNS, limit its usefulness.

Vector control

Tsetse fly control may be achieved by insecticide spraying, by modifying fly habitats, and by the trapping of flies. Reduction of man–fly contact by the felling of trees and vegetation around water contact points, so removing the shaded resting places of the tsetse fly, has proven to be a useful method of control of riverine species. Traps and screens impregnated with insecticide have been highly effective in reducing the riverine tsetse population in some areas. Selective spraying of residual insecticides on tsetse habitats is widely used. The control of the savannah tsetse however is generally not practicable. Aerial insecticide spraying of large areas has been employed but is costly and raises environmental concerns.

Reservoir elimination

In the past, sleeping sickness control campaigns have sometimes included destruction of wild game. This is not now considered either desirable or acceptable.

Manipulation of man's behaviour

The chronicity of gambiense disease means that its distribution through endemic areas is enhanced by the ability of infected persons to work and travel. Active case-finding and treatment is an important method of control, and to this and the development of more sensitive diagnostic tests with field application and the establishment of safer, more effective treatment regimens is essential. This approach is not helpful in the control of rhodesiense disease, a zoonosis with usually only sporadic human cases, unless an epidemic involving man–fly–man transmission occurs.

The promotion of agricultural development, or other forms of land use, encourages the destruction of tsetse habitats and the removal of game animals on which they feed. Individual protection can be achieved by the use of suitable insect repellents and insecticide impregnated clothing.

5

American Trypanosomiasis

American trypanosomiasis, widely known as Chagas' disease, is a protozoan parasitic infection caused by *Trypanosoma cruzi*. It is usually transmitted to man through breaks in the skin or mucous membrane contaminated with trypanosome infected faeces of the blood sucking 'cone-nosed' reduviid (triatomine) bug. The acute disease is characterized by fever, local oedematous swelling, lymphadenitis, myocarditis and occasionally meningoencephalitis. A chronic disease state with cardiomyopathy or the progressive development of megaoesophagus or megacolon may follow a latent period of asymptomatic infection.

EPIDEMIOLOGY

Human infection is widespread in rural areas and city slums in many parts of tropical and subtropical Central and South America including the Caribbean. The distribution of human *T. cruzi* in the Americas is determined by the behaviour of the vector bugs, the disease being endemic where the vectors are domestic dwellers. Most disease is found in northern Argentina, Bolivia, Paraguay, Uruguay, central coastal and southern Brazil and the southern half of Peru. Human disease is absent from the Amazon basin.

The parasite

The infective form of *T. cruzi* is the trypomastigote which circulates in the mammalian bloodstream and is ingested by the reduviid bug during the course of a blood meal.

Trypomastigotes are spindle-shaped organisms about 20 microns in length having an undulating membrane which arises from a posteriorly sited kinetoplast and extends along the entire length of the protozoan. The trypomastigotes transform into epimastigotes, or crithidial forms, within the bug's mid-gut and multiply extracellularly by binary fission. Crithidial forms are of similar size and shape as trypomastigotes but have a kinetoplast located anterior to the central nucleus and a short undulating membrane. Some 8 to 10 days after ingestion of trypomastigotes, and thereafter during the lifetime of the reduviid bug, metacyclic (slender) trypomastigote forms appear in the bug faeces. These are the forms infective to man and other mammalian hosts. Metacyclic trypomastigotes enter the wound made by the biting bug or are scratched into small skin abrasions. Trypomastigotes do not multiply in the blood but enter cells of mesenchymal origin, including cells of the reticuloendothelial system, myocardial cells and other smooth and striated muscle cells. They transform intracellularly into round or oval aflagellate leishmanial forms each measuring 3 to 5 microns in diameter. Here they multiply by binary fission until the cell ruptures and parasites are released to parasitize further host cells.

The vector

Blood sucking bugs belonging to the family *Reduviidae* are the vectors of *Trypanosoma cruzi*. These bugs are from 1–4 cm in length and have a snout-like head and prominent dark eyes. They have long lateral four-segmented antennae and a three-segmented proboscis which lies closely apposed to the ventral surface of the head. When the bug takes a blood meal it swings its proboscis downwards and forwards. The life cycle includes five nymphal stages, each resembling the adult, but lacking wings. Each nymphal stage requires a blood meal for further development. Nymphs and adults of both sexes feed on their hosts at night. Their bite is painless and each blood meal can take 25 minutes or more to complete. The bug defaecates whilst feeding and in doing so deposits trypomastigotes close to the bite wound, a habit facilitating the transmission of the parasite.

Reduviid bugs are widespread throughout Central and South America but human infection with *T. cruzi* has a patchy distribution and occurs in areas where the bugs are found in association with man's domestic habitat. Most species of reduviid bug are restricted to specialized sylvatic habitats, but some species, particularly *Triatoma infestans* (Brazil, Argentina, Chile, Peru), *Panstrongylus megistris* (Brazil) and *Rodnius prolixus* (Brazil, Venezuela, Colombia, Mexico) have adapted to a domestic or peridomestic habitat. Houses of poor construction offer good shaded conditions for the bugs to rest during the day. The distribution of bugs throughout buildings is governed by the ready availability of a blood meal and they tend to be found concentrated in the cracks and crevices of walls and roofs close to human sleeping areas and in buildings housing domestic animals. Adult bugs are capable of flying considerable distances in response to inadequate food supply, colonizing new habitats and so disseminating *T. cruzi* infection. Bugs breeding in palm trees attach their eggs to palm fronds. These bugs can be introduced into the domestic environment when these palm fronds are cut and used for house roofing. There have been suggestions that transmission of *T. cruzi* to man may result from contamination of food by the faeces of infected bugs and by ingestion of the bugs themselves.

Although vector-borne transmission accounts for the majority of cases of Chagas' disease, transmission both by blood transfusion and transplacentally contributes a small proportion of cases. *T. cruzi* has been demonstrated in maternal milk and it is believed transmission may occur during breast feeding.

Reservoir hosts

Chagas' disease is a zoonosis having both domestic and sylvatic reservoirs. Important sylvatic reservoirs include the opossum, anteater, armadillo and various forest primates. Dogs, cats, rats, guinea pigs and mice can all act as domestic reservoirs of disease. The link between the sylvatic and domestic cycles may be man (e.g. forestry workers) bringing infection from the forest to the domestic environment; wild animals straying into man's habitat; or bugs which, having been initially infected in the forest, are attracted to or carried into the house.

CLINICAL FEATURES

The acute phase of infection occurs within the first few weeks after inoculation with *T. cruzi* when trypomastigotes can usually be found on direct examination of peripheral blood. The majority of acute infections pass unnoticed being either asymptomatic or with trivial symptoms. In a small minority of cases, usually in children, a severe infection with a substantial mortality occurs.

At the site of penetration into the host the trypomastigotes invade surrounding cells, preferentially macrophages, and multiply locally producing a chagoma, which may appear as a granulomatous hyperpigmented scaly nodule at the portal of entry or, when infection occurs as a result of conjunctival entry, a periorbital oedematous swelling with tender local lymphadenopathy develops and often lasts for several weeks (Romana's sign). Dissemination of infection is by migrating parasitized macrophages, and by free trypomastigotes which appear in the blood 10 to 20 days after inoculation and cause the toxaemic phase of the illness. This is characterized by fever, generalized lymph node enlargement, hepatitis, splenomegaly, skin rashes, myocarditis and, occasionally, meningoencephalitis. Most such cases resolve after two to three months into a latent phase, which may remain asymptomatic, but is more likely to develop over a number of years into chronic Chagas' disease with clinical manifestations of cardiomyopathy or visceral dilatation. In the acute phase of the disease, myocardial insufficiency or severe meningoencephalitis are responsible for the 5 to 10% of cases which are fatal.

Chronic inflammation of the myocardium and smooth muscle of the gut, with infiltrates of lymphocytes and plasma cells, is the pathological basis of the chronic syndrome seen in Chagas' disease. In the acute phase of the disease inflammatory infiltrates in the myocardium are associated with amastigote nests but in chronic cases parasites cannot be found. It has been suggested that cardiac damage is secondary to an auto-immune phenomenon and that *T. cruzi* and heart muscle may share a common antigen.

Chagas' cardiomyopathy manifests itself in adult life between the ages of 15 and 50. The delay between initial infection and the clinical manifestations of cardiomyopathy ranges from 10 to 20 years. Cardiomyopathy is often asymptomatic and sudden death due to conduction defects may be its first manifestation. Investigation of patients known to have been infected with *T. cruzi* will often demonstrate electrocardiographic changes including various degrees of A-V block and primary ST-T wave changes. Cardiomyopathy may be present as chronic biventricular disease with predominantly right ventricular failure. Emboli from both right and left sides of the heart may cause pulmonary infarction and systemic embolization respectively.

Gastrointestinal manifestations of chronic Chagas' disease are mainly related to the progressive development of megaoesophagus or megacolon. A profound loss of autonomic ganglion cells from the intramural plexuses leads to characteristic distension and thinning of the walls of hollow viscera. Auto-immune cell destruction has been postulated as the mechanism for ganglion loss. Patients with megaoesophagus complain of increasing dysphagia, restrosternal discomfort and symptoms of overspill into the lungs. Megacolon is associated with severe constipation and faecal impaction, sigmoid volvulus and toxic megacolon.

The role of parasympathetic denervation producing other gastro-intestinal, endocrine or renal abnormalities remains to be determined. Chronic central and peripheral nervous system abnormalities have been described but not well defined.

The clinical picture of chronic Chagas' disease varies according to its geographical location and is related to the distribution of differing trypomastigote zymodemes. Cardiomyopathy is a prominent manifestation of disease in Venezuela, Columbia, southern Peru, and central and northern Chile. Megasyndromes are more commonly found in Paraguay, southern Brazil and northern Argentina.

DIAGNOSIS

The diagnosis of acute American trypanosomiasis depends upon isolation of *T. cruzi* from the blood, lymph node juice or rarely the cerebrospinal fluid, or its histological demonstration in lymph node, skin or muscle. In acute Chagas' disease, trypomastigotes of *T. cruzi* can regularly be found in the circulating blood on wet or Giemsa stained thick or thin blood films or in smears of the buffy coat. Trypomastigotes are not usually present in large numbers except in very young children during the acute early systemic phase. The parasites are fragile and easily damaged so that examination of freshly prepared specimens is necessary. Species identification of trypomastigotes is important, as man may also be infected with *T. rangeli*, a non-pathogen. *T. rangeli* has a very small rounded kinetoplast easily distinguished from the large oval kinetoplast in *T. cruzi*. In suspected Chagas' disease, blood films should be examined daily in the search for parasites. Trypanosomes may be present in the aspirated juice of lymph glands draining the site of the initial infection. In rare cases with clinical evidence of meningoencephalitis, *T. cruzi* can be isolated from the spun deposit of cerebrospinal fluid. Biopsy of a chagoma, an enlarged lymph gland or occasionally muscle in early Chagas' disease may reveal the presence of intracellular parasites in smears or histological sections stained with Romanowsky stains.

After the early toxic phase, trypomastigotes are not present in the blood in numbers detectable by microscopic techniques. Blood may be cultured on a suitable medium, e.g. Nicolle-Novy-McNeal, or by animal inoculation, in an attempt to demonstrate the organism.

In the technique of xenodiagnosis, laboratory bred bugs, free from *T. cruzi* infection, may be applied to the patient's skin in wire netting boxes and be permitted to take a blood meal. Pooled faeces from each box of bugs are then examined for metacyclic parasites after 30, 60 and 90 days. This is a time-consuming method and false negative results are not infrequent.

In the chronic illness, presumptive evidence from gastrointestinal radiography and electrocardiography should be supplemented by serological methods. Immunological diagnosis has been hampered by cross-reactions with antigens of *Leishmania* species and *T. rangeli*, but is currently being refined by use of purified antigens and their incorporation into enzyme-linked immunosorbent assays.

TREATMENT

Treatment of early toxaemic illness to diminish parasitaemia and minimize the risk of triggering auto-immune cardiomyopathy and ganglion cell death involves the use of relatively toxic drugs. Oral nifurtimox 10 mg/kg given daily (divided into three doses) for 60 days may cause gastrointestinal irritation, peripheral neuropathy and psychosis; whilst benznidiazole 5 mg/kg for 60 days causes polyneuritis, skin rashes and vomiting. Neither agent kills intracellular amastigotes or influences the chronic phase of illness, whose cardiac and gastrointestinal effects are treated on their own merits.

PREVENTION AND CONTROL

Vector control

Most preventative measures against Chagas' disease are directed against the domestic reduviid bug. Reduction of the population of bugs in human dwellings can be achieved by improvements in

Prevention and control 53

housing standards. House walls and floors can be plastered or cemented to eliminate cracks and crevices. Roofs made of palm thatch which provide shelter for bugs can be replaced with tiles or corrugated iron.

Insecticides are used for residual spraying inside houses and outbuildings. Regular application of insecticide and the participation of householders in vigilance schemes has proven to be a successful method of control.

Vector control programmes are limited by apathy and ignorance of householders, remoteness of many rural communities and by expense.

Reservoir elimination

Chemotherapeutic control by treatment of infected human cases is clearly not feasible when the majority of infected individuals have asymptomatic, latent disease.

The role of domestic animals as reservoirs of infection must be recognized and consideration given to their exclusion from the vicinity of houses.

Manipulation of man's behaviour

Health education has an important role in increasing public awareness of the problem and in encouraging community participation in control campaigns.

Sleeping under bed nets gives individual protection since the bugs only feed at night.

Transmission by blood transfusion can be reduced by serological screening of blood donors.

6
Amoebiasis

AETIOLOGY AND EPIDEMIOLOGY

Amoebic infection has a worldwide distribution. In man, several species of *Entamoeba* may be found in the lumen of the large bowel, but *Entamoeba histolytica* alone has undisputed pathogenicity. *Entamoeba* is a protozoon which normally lives in the contents of the large intestine, but can under certain circumstances become invasive. The infective form for man is the cyst which, when ingested, excysts in the small intestine releasing trophozoites which migrate to the large bowel. These motile trophozoites have a mean diameter of 20 µm and multiply by binary fission. Encystment of commensal trophozoites occurs as they pass down the colon, in response to adverse drier conditions in the local environment. Cysts are passed in the formed stools of carriers, as round or oval hyaline bodies, 10–20 µm in diameter. Each rigid-walled cyst contains up to four nuclei and is resistant to external environmental conditions. At normal environmental temperatures, amoebic cysts can survive for up to two weeks, and in cool water for several weeks. However, desiccation rapidly kills the cysts so that dust-borne infection is unlikely. Cysts are temperature sensitive and are killed by heating to above 50 °C and freezing below −5 °C.

Infection is often a consequence of urban overcrowding, poor sanitation, poverty and ignorance in a hot climate. Man becomes infected by ingesting cysts from faecal material either contaminating food or less often water, or spread directly from person to person. The main source of infection is the symptomless (non-dysenteric) carrier who passes large numbers of cysts, typically at irregular intervals. Amoebic trophozoites are not infective, being short-lived outside the body and unable to survive exposure to human digestive juices.

Lack of public sanitation with inadequate sewage disposal greatly facilitates disease transmission. Vegetables may be contaminated when 'night soil' containing amoebic cysts is used as fertilizer or polluted water used to freshen salads or soft fruit. Cysts survive passage through the digestive tracts of flies and cockroaches which along with cyst excreting food handlers are another source of amoebic infection.

Where levels of hygiene are low, direct contact with cyst containing human faeces may lead to household or institutional infection, but amoebic dysentery rarely occurs in epidemic form. Dogs and smaller mammals may be infected with *E. histolytica* but it is exceptional for them to be a source of infection for man as they do not pass faecal cysts.

Some strains of *E. histolytica* which carry the appropriate zymodemes may become invasive, causing host tissue necrosis and clinical disease. Commensal trophozoites appear sluggish with blunt pseudopodia and contain bacteria and other particles. Invasive trophozoites are more active with cytoplasmic vacuoles containing ingested host erythrocytes and cell fragments. Host factors that promote invasive amoebiasis include protein calorie malnutrition, impaired cellular immunity, systemic or local glucocorticoids, cytotoxic therapy, or pre-existing local disease including carcinoma and intestinal schistosomiasis.

The duration of *E. histolytica* infection varies widely, often persisting for two or three years. Spontaneous loss of infection is common but past infection does not appear to protect against reinfection or modify its severity.

CLINICAL FEATURES

Acute amoebic dysentery

Invasive bowel disease can occur anywhere in the large bowel and not infrequently affects its whole length. Sometimes it extends into the terminal ileum or involves the appendix. Initial lesions are usually located in the caecum or other sites of colonic stasis such as the flexures or rectosigmoid junction and disease may remain confined to one or more of these sites.

The earliest lesions are minute yellow nodules with surrounding hyperaemia which break down to small discrete mucosal erosions. Variably shaped ulcer craters form with a basal slough stained with faecal tissue. During the acute phase the ulcers enlarge and undermine the mucosa to give rise to 'collar stud' abscesses. The intervening mucosa is normal. Multiple ulcers may cause considerable oedematous thickening of the gut wall and in severe cases, the entire colonic mucosa may be ulcerated.

The muscularis mucosae is relatively resistant to amoebic infection but, in chronic disease or with marked secondary infection, it may be penetrated. Deep 'flask shaped' ulcers form with characteristic overhanging edges. If the tough muscularis externae is also breached, bowel perforation follows.

Healing of the mucosa occurs without scarring but where destruction of the muscularis mucosae has occurred, stricture of the colon may develop.

Blood vessels involved in the disease process may thrombose or bleed. Infarction necrosis of the bowel wall is thought to be one cause of transmural lesions which lead to colonic perforation and peritonitis. Bleeding from an arteriole is uncommon but may be severe and is sometimes fatal.

The incubation period of acute amoebic dysentery may be as short as 8 to 10 days or up to several months and may be difficult to determine, as overt disease may follow a prolonged asymptomatic infection or a variable period of minor abdominal symptoms.

The onset of amoebic dysentery is usually insidious with nausea, central gripping abdominal pain, which may be severe, and diarrhoea with up to 12 dysenteric motions daily. Low grade fever, toxaemia and abdominal distension are common. After an interval of a few days to several weeks, acute symptoms subside and the patient usually feels much better. There follows a variable period of remission, sometimes with constipation, before another attack of acute dysentery. This sequence may continue for many years.

Local acute complications of amoebic bowel disease include intestinal perforation and haemorrhage. When a major mesenteric vessel is eroded, massive sometimes fatal haemorrhage may result. Intestinal perforation occurs in up to 1% of amoebic bowel disease, most commonly in the caecum, ascending colon, sigmoid colon or rectum. It may be either acute or subacute, depending upon the degree to which peritoneal reaction has localized the spread of infection. Subacute perforation is associated with adhesion formation, pericolic abscesses, an inflammatory mass or retroperitoneal cellulitis.

Extra-intestinal complications usually occur some time after initial infection. Amoebic liver abscess and its sequelae are the most common, but abscesses may be found in other organs including the brain. Skin lesions including sinuses and ulcers arise usually by direct extension of colonic or liver disease.

Very occasionally cases may be fulminant with severe toxicity, swinging fever, prostration and dehydration, with up to 20 dysenteric watery motions daily. The faeces contain blood, mucus, flecks of faecal matter and large numbers of trophozoites, and sometimes gangrenous sloughs of the bowel wall. This condition may progress rapidly to meteorism, toxic megacolon and ileus and may be followed by widespread multiple bowel perforation and general peritonitis.

Post-dysenteric colitis may follow a severe attack of amoebic colitis. It is often refractory to treatment but resolves spontaneously.

Amoeboma

An amoeboma is a chronic localized amoebic infection of the wall of the large bowel which can develop months or years after the original infection. It occurs most commonly at sites of natural faecal stasis, the colonic flexures, caecum and rectosigmoid junction. The mucosal surface is usually ulcerated and covered by slough stained with faecal pigment and may extend for several centimetres. Histologically, an amoeboma consists of necrotic and oedematous granulation tissue with secondary fibrosis. Cellular elements include lymphocytes, plasma cells, eosinophils and rarely a few amoebic trophozoites may be distinguished.

An amoeboma may present as abdominal pain, change in bowel habit, intestinal colic, sub-acute intestinal obstruction or intussusception. A palpable abdominal mass may be present and may give rise to a differential diagnosis including a colonic carcinoma or an appendix mass. Fever may be present due to secondary bacterial infection of the amoeboma. An amoeboma is a late complication and does not give rise to trophozoites or cysts in the stool.

Amoebic liver abscess (ALA)

Trophozoites may enter the hepatic portal system and become lodged within intra-hepatic portal radicles. A proportion of these may die but in the presence of pre-existent liver disease, with the exception of cirrhosis, a number grow and multiply. Amoebic liver abscess does not usually present at the time of acute dysentery and may follow colonic infection by many years. Less than 50% of patients with ALA give a history of preceding dysentery. ALA is a condition of adults rather than children (10:1) and occurs more frequently in males than females (9:1).

Amoebic liver disease leads to focal destruction of liver cells, caused by proteolytic enzymes contained in *E. histolytica*. One or more foci of liver cell necrosis and liquefaction may coalesce and give rise to a single or, less frequently, to multiple abscesses, most commonly sited in the right lobe anteriorly below the diaphragm. Trophozoites are present in the shaggy ill-defined abscess wall and to a lesser extent in the sterile reddish-brown pus (consisting largely of lysed liver cells). Strictly these lesions are not true abscesses as they do not normally contain true pus. Secondary bacterial infection, however, may occur.

As it enlarges, the abscess becomes more sharply defined from surrounding tissues which are hyperaemic and oedematous with an inflammatory cell infiltrate. Biliary obstruction with jaundice is uncommon. Adhesions are formed with surrounding structures and organs as the eroding abscess mass approaches the liver surface, thereby reducing the likelihood of rupture. The abscess may however rupture into the abdomen, chest or onto the skin surface. Rarely, an abscess may erode a vein, when amoebae are carried in the blood to the brain and other organs.

An early symptom is often the feeling of heaviness, fullness or discomfort in the area of the liver. There develops local tenderness and often sharp stabbing right hypochondrial pain made worse by coughing. Moderate fever may develop, at first intermittent, then remittent and by the time an abscess forms there is often high swinging fever, profuse night sweats, rigors, intense continuous right hypochondrial discomfort and tenderness and right shoulder tip pain made worse by movement, deep breathing or coughing. The patient may notice a swelling in the right upper abdomen. Constitutional upset is prominent with rapidly progressive weight loss and anaemia.

The principal physical sign is an enlarged and tender liver, often with a point of maximum tenderness, and is sometimes associated with oedema over the lower ribs. When the abscess is deeply situated there may be little external evidence of abnormality but tenderness on hepatic percussion is then a valuable clinical sign. There may be a pleural rub, and crackles at the right lung base are common. Radiologically, localized elevation of the right hemidiaphragm may be seen with or without pulmonary collapse, consolidation or a pleural effusion.

An amoebic liver abscess enlarges progressively and may rupture into adjacent organs. Upward extension usually produces adhesions with the diaphragm and visceral pleura and a serous effusion at the right lung base is common. The abscess may rupture into the pleural space or more dramatically rupture into the lung giving rise to a hepatobronchial fistula resulting in expectoration of necrotic liver tissue, and occasionally flooding of the bronchial tree and death. Subphrenic rupture and rupture into the peritoneal cavity are less common. Extension into the pericardial sac may present as cardiac tamponade or with the more gradual onset of retrosternal chest pain with an associated pericardial friction rub. Rarely a large abscess compresses the common bile duct or several intrahepatic bile ducts causing obstructive jaundice. Less commonly, ALA leads to sinus formation and local skin amoebiasis, or fistulae may be formed with the gut, renal tract, a major blood vessel (e.g the inferior vena cava) or other organs. Blood-borne amoebic infection can spread to any organ including the lungs and brain. An abscess in the brain may produce symptoms of a space occupying lesion but is often silent.

Skin lesions

Amoebic skin ulceration may develop around the anus, colostomy stomata or surgical laparotomy scars as direct extensions from large bowel disease, or in the skin surrounding sinuses which may develop from an externally ruptured amoebic liver abscess.

Anogenital amoebiasis is a common form of the infection in Papua New Guinea and can give rise to balanitis, vulvitis, vaginitis and cervicitis.

DIAGNOSIS

Amoebic dysentery

The stool in acute amoebic dysentery contains loose faecal material and glutinous stringy mucus admixed with dark, semifluid blood. Stool microscopy will demonstrate numerous bacilli, red cells and amoebic trophozoites with ingested blood cells. Diagnosis of amoebic bowel disease requires identification of living haematophagous (erythrocyte containing) trophozoites of *E. histolytica* in freshly passed stool, bowel wall scrapings or colonic biopsy material obtained at sigmoidoscopy or colonoscopy.

Trophozoites tend to be clumped or massed together in the mucus and are not evenly distributed in a stool sample. Examination of fresh stool is required. Trophozoites will round up and cease movement within 15 minutes of cooling, making their identification extremely difficult.

The finding of non-haematophagous trophozoites and/or cysts of *E. histolytica* in the stool in the presence of dysentery must not be regarded as evidence of causation. In carriers, cysts are found in the faecal part of the stool and concentration methods are often necessary for their isolation and identification. In stool emulsified with 1% eosin cysts stand out as round or oval white objects against a pink background. In stool prepared with Lugol's iodine solution the cysts are recognized by their iodine stained nuclei and glycogen vacuoles. It is usual to examine at least three stool concentrates from samples obtained at intervals, as cysts tend to appear intermittently. Cysts of *E. histolytica* can be distinguished from those of other amoebae on the basis of size and number of nuclei present. Cysts of *E. histolytica* contain four nuclei (occasionally less when immature) and have a mean diameter greater than 10 μm. Faeces that cannot be examined fresh for trophozoites or cysts should be preserved in merthiolate-iodine-formalin or polyvinyl alcohol. Staining techniques are available to enable identification of trophozoites from these preparations.

The differential diagnosis of amoebic dysentery includes bacillary dysentery, ulcerative colitis, intestinal salmonellosis and schistosomiasis. Distinction between acute amoebiasis and bacillary dysentery is in most cases straightforward. The patient with amoebiasis is usually ambulant and acute prostration and dehydration are rare.

Radiological investigation is rarely helpful in the diagnosis of uncomplicated amoebic colitis, but barium studies may be utilized in the diagnosis of an amoeboma or stricture. Sigmoidoscopy may be required to obtain material for examination if trophozoites are not found in the stool. The commonest findings in amoebic colitis are small submucous haemorrhages covered with flecks of blood-stained mucus in which trophozoites can be found. Less commonly shallow ulcers with a yellow exudate are seen. Material for examination from these ulcers can be obtained by gentle scraping with a Volkmann spoon.

Amoebic liver abscess

An amoebic liver abscess is usually associated with a polymorph leukocytosis and a normocytic hypochromic or normochromic anaemia. Liver function tests often reveal normal transaminases and modest elevation of alkaline phosphatase and gamma-glutamyl transferase levels; that is, the pattern of a space-occupying lesion. Trophozoites and cysts are usually absent from the stools.

A chest radiograph may show local upward bulging or 'tenting' of the right hemi-diaphragm and screening indicate a lack of movement with respiration. Both pleural reaction or effusion and pulmonary shadowing or collapse are often seen at the right lung base. Other investigations with particular localizing value include radioisotope liver scanning, ultrasound and computerized axial tomography. It is of note that ultrasonic evidence of the presence of a liver abscess often remains for a considerable time after cure.

Percutaneous needle aspiration of lesions in the liver may rarely be necessary for diagnostic purposes. The finding of trophozoites in the pus, usually taken from the last of the aspirate, is diagnostic. Indications for aspiration of liver abscesses are impending rupture and the failure of the abscess to resolve on drug therapy alone.

The differential diagnosis of amoebic liver abscess includes hepatic malignancy, commonly primary hepatoma in the tropics, or secondary carcinoma. Pyogenic liver abscess is usually of a more acute onset than amoebic abscess, whilst hydatid disease of the liver is more insidious in onset, and differentiated from ALA by ultrasound examination.

Amoebic serology

A number of serological tests have been used to assist in the diagnosis of amoebiasis. The most sensitive methods include ELISA, indirect immunofluorescence, indirect agglutination, and counter immunoelectrophoresis. These tests fail to distinguish between past and present infection, and in endemic areas many people give positive results, although usually at low titres. Using sensitive tests over 95% of patients with liver abscess are positive, as are between 60–80% with invasive bowel disease. Their main value is that when negative this is strong evidence against a diagnosis of amoebiasis. Most serological tests remain positive long after successful treatment and are of little value in assessing cure. The gel diffusion precipitin test is often the first serological test to revert to normal after cure.

TREATMENT

The aim of treatment is to eradicate all *E. histolytica* organisms, both in the tissues and bowel lumen. Anti-amoebic drugs have been classified as either tissue (systemic) or lumenal amoebicides, depending upon their site of action. Tissue amoebicides kill invasive trophozoites but may have little effect upon non-invasive trophozoites and cysts and relapse may follow treatment of amoebic dysentery when a tissue amoebicide is used alone. In non-endemic areas, at least five negative stool tests carried out over four weeks after completion of a course of treatment are needed to prove parasitological cure.

Drug therapy

Metronidazole
Both metronidazole and tinidazole are effective in all types of amoebiasis. Metronidazole is a potent and safe tissue amoebicide and is to a lesser extent useful as a lumenal amoebicide. These drugs are the treatment of choice for amoebic colitis, amoeboma, liver abscess and for preoperative medication for bowel surgery in the presence of amoebic infection. Metronidazole is less useful in the treatment of asymptomatic cyst passers. Adverse side-effects of metronidazole include gastrointestinal upset, nausea, vomiting, diarrhoea, headache, skin rash, stomatitis, a metallic taste in the mouth, transient ataxia and intolerance of alcohol. Prolonged courses can cause leukopenia and peripheral neuropathy. Metronidazole has been used widely in pregnancy without evidence of foetal damage.

Emetine hydrochloride
Emetine hydrochloride and dihydroemetine are highly effective tissue amoebicides but are now less used than formerly. Emetine hydrochloride is the most potent tissue amoebicide, while dihydroemetine is thought to be less cumulative and cardiotoxic but

neither can be given orally in view of their immediate stimulus to vomiting. Neither are effective against amoebic cysts within the gut. Myocardial toxicity is the most serious problem with emetine, especially with intravenous administration and intramuscular or deep subcutaneous injection is advisable. Even so, patients should be kept rested and under cardiological observation during and for a time after treatment.

Antibiotics
Tetracycline is an indirect-acting lumenal amoebicide effective through its antibacterial properties. Tetracycline should be avoided during pregnancy and in young children. Erythromycin has a greater direct amoebicidal action and is safe to use in infants and young children.

Diloxanide furoate
Diloxanide furoate (Furamide) is a safe and useful lumenal amoebicide commonly prescribed alone for treatment of asymptomatic cyst passers or with metronidazole in amoebic dysentery. Absorption from the gut is poor. Adverse side-effects include occasional nausea and flatulence.

Treatment of amoebic dysentery

The treatment of choice is metronidazole given in doses of 800 mg three times daily along with Furamide 500 mg three times daily, both for a period of 5 days. Metronidazole at this dosage may cause nausea and vomiting and a lower dose of 400 mg three times daily for 5 days with Furamide 500 mg three times daily for ten to 20 days may be preferred. The lower dose of metronidazole will effect prompt clinical cure, but the prolonged course of Furamide is required for complete eradication of the amoebae.

In severe cases tetracycline 500 mg three times daily for 5 days along with either emetine hydrochloride 65 mg or dihydroemetine 100 mg given daily intramuscularly or subcutaneously until diarrhoea subsides may be given as additional treatment.

Paediatric doses are less than those given for adults.

Treatment of amoeboma

Metronidazole is effective in amoeboma. Any delay in resolution should raise the possibility of other or associated pathology, particularly carcinoma.

Treatment of amoebic liver abscess

Metronidazole in a dose of 400 mg three times daily for 10 days is the standard treatment for ALA. With large abscesses and those threatening rupture therapeutic aspiration should be considered. Failure to improve after five days of treatment with metronidazole is also an indication for aspiration of the abscess. Dramatic improvement will often follow this procedure. An attempt to aspirate the abscess to dryness must be made and meticulous aseptic technique adopted.

Most patients with ALA no longer have a patent lumenal infection and there is no evidence to suggest a role for lumenal amoebicides.

Treatment of brain abscess

Response to medication including emetine is poor and the condition is almost always fatal.

Treatment of carriers

In temperate climates all carriers of amoebiasis should be treated to eliminate the infection. In the tropics and areas where amoebiasis is endemic, it is usual to treat asymptomatic carriers in certain categories only, notably food handlers and those who have recently suffered invasive disease, to prevent relapse. Furamide, the lumenal amoebicide, is prescribed in a dosage of 500 mg orally three times daily for 10 days. Paediatric dosage is 20 mg/kg body weight daily in three divided doses.

PREVENTION AND CONTROL

Travellers to endemic areas should avoid uncooked foods and unboiled water (boiling for 5 minutes kills cysts). Salads and soft fruits grown close to the ground and perhaps fertilized with night soil should be soaked in diluted sodium hypochlorite solution or potassium permanganate solution for 30 minutes and then rinsed in boiled water.

Community measures to control spread of amoebiasis include provision or improvement of piped water and services for sewage disposal. Chlorination of water does not destroy amoebic cysts which are removed by filtration. Water likely to contain cysts should be treated with a coagulant and allowed to settle before filtration. In practice, control of amoebiasis has proved difficult in highly endemic areas.

7
Giardiasis

AETIOLOGY AND EPIDEMIOLOGY

Giardia lamblia is a flagellated protozoon that was first discovered by Leeuwenhoek in 1681, who found the parasite in his own stools, but was properly described by Lambl in 1859. There are believed to be over 40 species of *Giardia*. *Giardia lamblia*, the species known to infect man, also naturally infects beaver, cattle, cat and dog. *Giardia muris* infects primarily mice and rats and *G. agilis* is found in amphibians.

The trophozoite of *G. lamblia* is a motile flagellate which is found in the small intestine, in particular the duodenum and upper jejunum. It is from 9 to 21 μm long and 5 to 15 μm wide, with a convex dorsal surface and a flat ventral surface containing a circular 'sucking' disc. They are most numerous at the bases of the microvilli where they attach themselves to the mucosa via their ventral disc and sometimes become superficially invasive. Nourishment is obtained by diffusion through the cell wall.

Infection in man follows the ingestion of viable cysts of *G. lamblia*. The infectious dose is believed to be as low as ten cysts. The protozoa excysts in the stomach and upper small intestine. Persons with achlorhydria, hypogammaglobulinaemia, (particularly low levels of IgA), and with acquired immunodeficiency syndrome are particularly susceptible to infection.

The trophozoite can divide by binary fission every 5 to 10 hours. The incubation period in man is usually 1 to 3 weeks and infection lasts, if untreated, for 4 to 6 weeks but may be more chronic. Symptomless carriage is common, symptoms occurring in as few as 20% of infections.

Factors that lead to release of the trophozoite and to encystment are not clear. Cysts are thin walled and oval in shape measuring 8–12 μm in length and 7 to 12 μm in width and contain two to four nuclei and refractile fibrils. The number of cysts found in the stool does not necessarily reflect the intensity of infection. Variable numbers of cysts are often passed in a cyclical fashion. In patients with watery diarrhoea and a rapid transit time, trophozoites may be found in the stool.

Giardiasis is commonest where sanitation is poor, the highest incidence being found in the tropics. Many recent reports have confirmed its occurrence in temperate zones and it is now the most commonly reported protozoan parasite worldwide. In areas where giardiasis is common the incidence appears to be highest in children, reflecting the fact that it is most commonly spread by the faecal–oral route. Direct person-to-person spread can be a particular problem in children's institutions. In the tropics giardiasis is a family infection with person-to-person spread by faecal–oral infection from hand feeding in poor hygienic conditions. Water-borne transmission is common and cysts can be found in sewage effluent, in surface waters and in some potable water supplies. Occasionally giardiasis may occur in epidemic form in developed countries, associated with contamination of water supplies. Contamination of streams and rivers by animal reservoirs such as beavers has led to infection in campers. Food-borne outbreaks have been documented in the developed world and in the rural tropics vegetables contaminated by using human excreta as fertilizer are often the vehicle of infection.

CLINICAL FEATURES

The parasite is a common cause of diarrhoeal illness both in the tropics and in temperate zones. Infection with giardia can give rise to an acute, self-limiting illness, characterized by the sudden onset of explosive, foul-smelling watery diarrhoea that is free of blood and pus. There is abundant intestinal gas manifested by abdominal distension, foul-smelling flatulence and belching. Upper abdominal cramping pains, anorexia and nausea are common and vomiting occurs in some patients. Systemic features may include generalized weakness and low grade fever. Weight loss is not uncommon. Initial watery diarrhoea may give way to greasy frothy stools and varying degrees of malabsorption.

The duration of the acute clinical illness varies widely. Some patients have a short-lived illness whilst in others the illness persists for months. The acute infection commonly resolves spontaneously and the parasite disappears from the faeces. Some patients become asymptomatic carriers for a period of time after the acute illness, occasionally developing a recurrence of symptoms. Sometimes infection persists giving rise to chronic malabsorption, steatorrhoea and marked loss of weight. Host factors, in particular the immune response, and differences in strain virulence are probably important factors in determining the severity of disease. The mechanism by which giardia produces diarrhoea and malabsorption has not been clearly established. Mucosal injury secondary to inflammatory changes along with lumenal factors such as bacterial overgrowth with bile salt deconjugation and bile salt depletion (secondary to significant uptake into the parasitic cytoplasm) may be contributory factors.

DIAGNOSIS

The principal method of diagnosis is by demonstration of the organism in faecal specimens or material from the small intestine. Both trophozoites and cysts can be identified on direct smears of stools or following concentration techniques. Diarrhoeal specimens should be examined within one hour after being passed or should be preserved in polyvinyl alcohol (PVA) or a 10% formalin solution as trophozoites are unstable outside the gastrointestinal tract. Formed stools, which are more likely to contain the more hardy cysts, can be examined within 24 hours or longer if refrigerated or placed in fixative. Identification is usually performed using a direct wet mount preparation on a concentrated stool sample. Permanent staining of the faecal sample may improve detection rates.

Stool examination may be negative in the early stages of infection and in patients who shed organisms in a cyclical pattern. The collection of three separate stools, one collected every second or third day, will improve the detection rate to 90%. Medications, including antibiotics, antacids and antidiarrhoeal compounds, along with barium used in radiological studies, can interfere with identification of the organism by altering its morphology or by causing a temporary disappearance of parasites from stool specimens.

Patients suspected of having giardiasis but with negative stool results may have trophozoites in the upper small intestine which can be demonstrated in intestinal fluid or biopsy. Upper intestinal fluid can be sampled endoscopically or by using the 'sticky string' test. An intestinal biopsy may be examined by staining touch smears or tissue sections.

Countercurrent immunoelectrophoresis, enzyme-linked immunosorbent assays and DNA probes have been developed to detect giardia antigen in stool specimens and can be more sensitive than stool microscopy. As a research tool serological testing can demonstrate an early specific anti-giardia IgM response which if present is highly suggestive of active infection. Detecting an anti-giardia IgG response, however, does not distinguish current from past exposure to the parasite.

Demonstration of the parasite is not conclusive proof of causal association with symptoms and other infections or enteropathies may lead to the chance recognition of previously undetected carriage of the parasite.

When specifically tested, patients often have laboratory evidence of malabsorption with lactase deficiency, abnormal D-xylose excretion and abnormal vitamin B_{12} absorption.

TREATMENT

The drug of choice for the treatment of giardiasis is one of the imidazole drugs. Metronidazole in a single 2.0 g dose for three successive days produced a parasitological cure in 91% of patients. Children age 1–3 years should be given 500 mg daily; age 3–7 years 600–800 mg daily; and 7–10 year olds 1.0 g daily for 3 days. Side-effects of metronidazole include a metallic taste, headaches, nausea and a disulfiram-like effect with alcohol. Metronidazole is sometimes better tolerated in adults in a dose of 400 mg three times daily for 5 days. Tinidazole in a single dose of 2.0 g is probably as effective and appears to have fewer side-effects than metronidazole. Relapses are uncommon but can occur up to 6 months after treatment.

Continuing symptoms after treatment may be as a result of lactase deficiency secondary to damage to the mucosal brush border or secondary pathology. Frequent relapses may occur in the immunodeficient. The treatment of asymptomatic cyst carriers in an endemic area may be non-productive unless treatment is being given as part of a wider control programme.

PREVENTION AND CONTROL

Control in endemic areas in the developing world will depend upon the provision of a clean water supply and improved sanitation. Personal protection involves the avoidance of uncooked vegetables and untreated water. Cysts can withstand chlorination at concentrations used to disinfect water, but are susceptible to heat and to prolonged freezing.

8
Cryptosporidiosis

AETIOLOGY AND EPIDEMIOLOGY

Cryptosporidiosis is widely distributed in the tropics and is a cause of diarrhoeal disease particularly in children, and in patients with AIDS.

Cryptosporidium is a coccidian protozoon, 2–5 μm in diameter, that parasitizes epithelium. Oocysts are ingested in contaminated food or water, or by direct transmission via the faecal–oral route. A very small dose, probably less than ten organisms, is required to cause disease. In the small bowel the oocysts sporulate, excyst and release infective sporozoites that adhere to enterocyte surfaces, becoming enclosed in a parasitophorous vacuole. The parasite thus becomes intracellular but extracytoplasmic. A complete development cycle occurs within a single host.

In the immunocompetent the parasite is usually confined to the bowel, with the ileum being most heavily colonized. In immunocompromised hosts, infection extends to epithelial surfaces outside the gut, e.g. gall bladder, bile and pancreatic ducts, pharynx, oesophagus, bronchi and sinuses. Pathological changes include epithelial cell loss, villous atrophy, crypt elongation, and minimal inflammatory changes in the lamina propria.

CLINICAL FEATURES

After an incubation period of 2 to 14 days there is onset of illness with watery diarrhoea, which may be associated with nausea and vomiting, abdominal pain, malaise, myalgias and fever. The diarrhoea is self-limiting in normal hosts and is of 10 to 14 days (range 1 to 60 days) duration.

In immunocompromised hosts diarrhoea is often intractable. Patients experience frequent, large volume, episodes of diarrhoea, leading to severe dehydration, malabsorption and profound weight loss, the so-called 'slim' disease of Uganda. Patients with AIDS and cryptosporidiosis may have biliary tract involvement. In these patients nausea, vomiting and abdominal pain, often localized to the right upper quadrant, are more pronounced.

DIAGNOSIS

The diagnosis depends on identification of oocysts in faecal smears. A modified acid-fast stain is commonly used. Parasites can also be identified in biopsy specimens, e.g. small intestine, and less commonly rectum. Examination of duodenal aspirate is reported to be more sensitive than stool examination.

TREATMENT

There is no effective specific therapy. Treatment depends upon adequate fluid and electrolyte replacement and nutritional support.

PREVENTION AND CONTROL

Control requires special emphasis on personal hygiene and sanitary disposal of faeces. The parasite is resistant to many disinfectants, including the concentration of chlorine and iodine usually used to disinfect water.

Part Two
Helminthiases

9
Roundworm Diseases

ASCARIASIS

Aetiology and epidemiology

It is estimated that one in four of the world's population is infected with *Ascaris lumbricoides*, most of these belonging to the developing countries of the tropics and subtropics. To illustrate the extent of the worm burden it has been estimated that if all *Ascaris* were placed head to tail they would span the world 50 times; or put another way 1000 tons of *Ascaris* exist at any one time.

This large roundworm, averaging 25 cm in length, lives in the small intestine of man. Each day the female worm produces in the order of 200 000 large, thick-shelled eggs which are able to survive in the environment for months and even years. The eggs are disseminated under insanitary conditions where there is indiscriminate defaecation and where human faeces are used as fertilizer – so-called 'night soil'. Under the right environmental conditions larvae develop within the eggs, which become infective within 3 to 4 weeks. Infection occurs when these embryonated eggs are ingested.

Eggs hatch in the jejunum, larvae penetrate the mucosa, and are carried via the bloodstream through the liver and heart to the lungs. Within the lung they escape from the capillaries into the alveoli and travel via the trachea and larynx into the pharynx to be swallowed and arrive again in the small intestine – a migration which lasts about 14 days. Over a period of 2 to 3 months there is development into mature adults. Adult worms have a lifespan of up to 2 years.

Clinical features

Migration of *Ascaris lumbricoides* larvae from the intestine to the liver and lungs usually occurs without clear symptoms unless the parasite load is heavy, when they may give rise to Loeffler's pneumonitis (see below).

Symptoms of intestinal infection vary from none through mild to acute colicky pain with distension, depending on the worm load. Intestinal obstruction, volvulus and intussusception by worm masses are important complications leading to up to 100 000 deaths per year. Worms have a tendency to migrate from the small intestine, this occurring more commonly when they are 'stressed' by for example a febrile illness or administration of a general anaesthetic to the host. Worms may invade the ampullary orifice giving rise to biliary obstruction or acute pancreatitis. Ectopic worms can also lead to appendicitis, perforation of the bowel, and migration through operative suture lines causing peritonitis.

The contribution of ascaris infection to malnutrition is controversial. There is conflicting evidence as to whether or not the worms are a cause of malabsorption or whether they consume significant calories or essential elements in the diet. They can however reduce the appetite of a child and in this way contribute to protein energy malnutrition.

Loeffler's pneumonitis

The essential features of this syndrome are transitory, migratory pulmonary shadows associated with a peripheral eosinophilia. This may be asymptomatic, but the majority of patients experience symptoms of wheeze and cough, sometimes productive of yellow sputum which contains an abundance of eosinophilis. A few patients are febrile and suffer general malaise. The syndrome may develop as part of an allergic reaction to a number of drugs but is also recognized as a reaction to parasitic infection when there is a migratory phase in the parasitic life cycle. The list of parasites which may give rise to Loeffler's syndrome includes *Ascaris*, hookworm, *Trichuris*, *Trichinella*, *Taenia* and *Strongyloides*. Treatment is that of the causal agent.

Diagnosis

The microscopic detection of faecal eggs remains the best and simplest method of diagnosis. The eggs are round or oval in shape, brown in colour due to staining with bile pigments, and they measure some 60 µm in length and 45 µm in breadth. There are several immunological diagnostic methods being developed. In the stage of larval migration there is a high eosinophilia, but eosinophilia is not a feature of adult infections.

Treatment

Pyrantel pamoate (Combantrin), given as a single dose of 10 mg/kg body weight, is inexpensive, has the advantage of single dose treatment, and is extremely effective against *Ascaris*. It does not however have a broad spectrum of activity against other helminths. Mebendazole (Vermox) is effective in a dose of 100 mg twice daily for 3 days. Mebendazole in addition to the disadvantage of multiple dosage is also unsuitable for pregnant women and children under 2 years of age, but has the advantage of being active against hookworm and *Trichuris*. Albendazole in a single dose of 400 mg is effective against *Ascaris* and has a broad spectrum of anti-helminthic activity. Levamisole as a single 4 mg/kg dose is effective, inexpensive and has been used successfully in mass treatment campaigns. Nausea and vomiting occur in about 1% of those treated.

Where a mass of worms has led to intestinal obstruction, drug therapy combined with intravenous fluids and the judicious use of liquid paraffin may lead to explusion of the worms and resolution of the obstruction. Surgical treatment should always be preceded by a trial of medical treatment whenever possible. It may be possible to milk the mass of worms into the large intestine, so avoiding a suture line and possible post-operative disruption and peritonitis by migrating worms overlooked at operation. A counsel of perfection in areas endemic for ascariasis would be to treat pre-operatively all patients requiring elective bowel surgery for potential infection.

Prevention and control

In many of the worst affected areas the enormous egg producing capacity of the worm combined with poor sanitation, cultural practices and inadequate financial resources prevent any serious attempt at control. Measures including the proper disposal of faeces and prevention of soil contamination in areas immediately adjacent to houses, particularly in children's play areas, composting of fertilizers to destroy eggs and other methods of protecting food from contamination should be instituted. Selective mass treatment of children has been successful in reducing the worm load.

HOOKWORM DISEASE

Aetiology and epidemiology

Hookworm disease is widespread in the tropics and subtropics. In man two species of hookworm are described: *Ancylostoma duodenale* and *Necator americanus*. *Necator americanus*, as the name implies, is widespread in the Americas, but is also commonly found in sub-Saharan Africa, South Asia and the Pacific. *Ancylostoma duodenale* is predominantly a parasite of southern Europe, north Africa, India and the East. There is considerable overlap in the distribution of the two species.

The adult worms, which measure some 1 cm by 0.5 cm, live in the jejunum and less commonly the duodenum of man. They attach themselves to the mucosa by their mouthparts and feed on blood. The female deposits eggs into the lumen of the small bowel. The daily output of eggs for the female *Necator americanus* is about 3000 whilst 15 000 to 20 000 eggs are produced daily by *Ancylostoma duodenale*. Eggs are passed in the faeces and in moist, warm, shady conditions the eggs hatch in the soil into rhabditiform larvae. These larvae feed on bacteria and moult twice to give rise to infective filariform larvae. These larvae require a human host in which to develop, and gain access to this host by penetrating the skin. The interdigital spaces of the bare-footed host are a favoured site of penetration. The larvae enter the venules and are carried via the right heart to the lungs. Once in the lung capillaries the larvae penetrate the capillary wall and enter the alveoli. They migrate up the trachea and into the pharynx from where they are swallowed, eventually reaching the small intestine where they attach to the mucosa and begin to feed. The worms become sexually mature in 3 to 5 weeks. The adult *A. duodenale* usually survives for a year (there have been reports of 5 to 7 years), whilst *N. americanus* can survive for 2 to 6 years (reports of 15 to 20 years).

Clinical features

Itchy papules may appear at the site of larval penetration, but are rarely recognized. The larvae, during their migratory phase in the lungs, may give rise to symptoms of cough and wheeze, but symptoms are only ever mild. Chest radiography may reveal transient pulmonary infiltrates.

The majority of hookworm infections are light and asymptomatic. Hookworm disease develops when the worm load is large and consequently blood loss and degree of anaemia is greatest. Each *A. duodenale* can cause loss of 0.2 ml of blood per day, the loss from *N. americanus* being less at 0.05 ml per day. The relative longevity of the worms combined with the not inconsiderable daily blood loss they create gives rise to an insidious and often profound iron deficiency anaemia. Because of its insidious development patients may have well compensated anaemias with haemoglobins of less than 5 g/dl and only present when their haemoglobin has dropped below this level and symptoms of tiredness, breathlessness and oedema have developed. Albumin loss is only significant in very heavy infections and oedema is secondary to the iron deficiency and sometimes a degree of heart failure.

Diagnosis

Finding the characteristic eggs in a direct stool smear will help establish the diagnosis of hookworm disease. The eggs are oval with a thin, transparent, colourless shell, and measure 60 μm by 40 μm. When freshly passed the egg contains a two to eight-segmented ovum. Stool concentration techniques are not appropriate, for if there are too few eggs to see on direct smear then the infection, if present, is insignificant, and not the cause of the anaemia. Where hookworm is common then eggs will often be found in stool. Every effort should be made to exclude other causes of iron deficiency before hookworm anaemia is diagnosed. Eosinophilia is often present and is maximal during the phase of tissue migration.

Treatment

In an endemic area, if hookworm infection is light and not causing anaemia, there is little indication to treat it, unless treatment forms part of a mass treatment control programme.

Albendazole is probably the drug of choice. A single dose of 400 mg will produce an 80% reduction in egg count and 200 mg daily for 3 days will give 100% cure. Albendazole is effective against both *N. americanus* and *A. duodenale*, as well as being active against *Ascaris*, and is therefore eminently suitable for mass treatment programmes. Pyrantel pamoate (Combantrin) can be used in a single dose of 10 mg/kg and is also effective against *Ascaris*. Mebendazole, 100 mg/kg twice daily for three days, is effective, as is Levimasole in a single 2.5 mg/kg single dose, although Levimasole appears to be less effective when treating *N. americanus*.

The iron deficiency should be treated with ferrous sulphate 400 mg two or three times daily. Treatment should be continued for three months after restoration of haemoglobin levels to allow for iron store replenishment. Consideration should be given to supplementation of vitamin B_{12} and folic acid in patients on a nutritional knife-edge, bearing in mind the massive and often rapid production of new red cells that has to take place.

Prevention and control

Health education with particular emphasis on safe disposal of faeces and the wearing of shoes in endemic areas is appropriate but often unsuccessful. Single dose treatments allow mass treatment campaigns. By regularly reducing the worm burden the haemoglobin levels and health of a population would be expected to increase.

Cutaneous larva migrans

Cutaneous larva migrans is a cutaneous eruption resulting from exposure of the skin to the infective filariform larvae of non-human hookworms, e.g. *A. braziliense*, a hookworm of cats and dogs, *A. caninum*, a dog hookworm, and various non-human *Strongyloides*. The infective larvae of these species penetrate the skin of man but on finding themselves in an inappropriate host are unable to develop and wander around under the skin. They can survive for many months before they eventually perish. Infection is acquired when skin comes into contact with damp contaminated soil. The feet are a common portal of entry but infection often occurs in the buttocks and trunk in those exposed to contaminated sand on coastal beaches. A small itchy papule develops at the portal of entry. Each larva can move up to several centimetres a day and leaves behind an intensely itchy, serpiginous track which when scratched may become secondarily infected. In contrast to the larva currens of *Strongyloides stercoralis* (see below) the tract is persistent and indurated with little or no surrounding flare.

Topical thiabendazole is the treatment of choice. It is given by grinding up a 0.5 g tablet with 5 g of petroleum jelly and applied liberally over the tract of the worm, and in particular the leading edge, daily for 5 days. Alternatively, thiabendazole can be given orally in a dose of 25 mg/kg twice daily for 5 days. Symptoms of itching usually resolve within 24 hours and the track heals within 7 to 14 days.

Cutaneous larva migrans can also be treated by local freezing of the head of the advancing track using an ethyl chloride spray.

STRONGYLOIDIASIS

Aetiology and epidemiology

Strongyloides stercoralis has a worldwide distribution in the tropics and subtropics, and is particularly prevalent in South-east Asia and parts of Brazil and Columbia.

The adult female worm is slender, 2 mm in length and found in the small intestine of man living embedded in the mucosa. A male worm exists but is not as yet identified. The female lays her eggs in the mucosa where they hatch into rhabditiform larvae. Eggs are not released into the bowel lumen and not therefore found in the stool. Rhabditiform larvae are however present in the faeces, and if they come to find themselves released into a warm, moist environment, will develop within a week into free-living male and female larvae. The larvae sexually reproduce to produce a new generation of free-living rhabditiform larvae and this cycle may be repeated many times. Under unfavourable environmental conditions the larvae will however develop into infective filariform forms. The filariform larvae can survive several weeks awaiting an opportunity to infect man, usually by penetrating the skin, though infection may also take place via the buccal mucosa from ingestion of food contaminated with infective larvae. After penetration the larvae are carried to the lungs, penetrate through into the alveoli, enter the bronchi, cross over the glottis and pass to the small intestine where they mature into adults within four weeks. Larvae may develop into infective filariform forms whilst still in the host's intestinal tract, and are able to reinfect the same host by either penetrating the bowel wall or perianal skin. In this way infection, once established, can be maintained within a single host for many years.

Clinical features

The larvae penetrating the skin may cause dermatitis with pruritis and urticaria. If the infecting dose is large, pulmonary symptoms may follow the migration through the lungs. Adult females sometimes develop and produce eggs in the lungs, and large numbers of larvae may then appear in the sputum. The adult worms in the small intestine may give rise to upper abdominal discomfort and diarrhoea, and frank steatorrhoea may occur with early *Strongyloides* infection. Symptoms usually subside within a few weeks and the infection becomes asymptomatic. During the course of this chronic infection bouts of intermittent diarrhoea may occur. Migration of larvae through the skin during auto-infection may give rise to a red, often serpiginous, evanescent, itchy eruption which is usually confined to the trunk and thighs. This 'larva currens' appears in crops at irregular and unpredictable intervals.

In immunocompromised hosts *Strongyloides* can disseminate widely throughout the body, causing serious and often fatal infection. There is usually severe diarrhoea, often with malabsorption, and paralytic ileus may develop. Severe dyspnoea caused by pulmonary larval infiltration is a common accompaniment. The migrating *Strongyloides* carry with them bowel flora, and Gram-negative septicaemia and pyogenic meningitis are frequent causes of death.

Diagnosis

Larvae may be identified in stool. In a patient with diarrhoea adult worms may be passed. Stool examination is, however, a poorly sensitive test. Microscopy of duodenal contents obtained by aspiration, biopsy or the hairy sticky string test (Enterotest capsules) gives an improved diagnostic yield.

Marked eosinophilia is common in strongyloidiasis but may be absent in patients who are on steroids or who are otherwise severely immunosuppressed. There is never an eosinophilia in the hyperinfection syndrome, all eosinophils having been used up in attempting to control the migrating larvae.

An ELISA using larval antigen has recently been developed and has both high sensitivity and specificity.

Treatment

Thiabendazole is effective in a dose of 25 mg/kg twice daily for 3 days, but will fail to eradicate infection in up to one third of patients. Albendazole 400 mg daily is at least as effective as thiabendazole and may prove to be the drug of choice.

For the treatment of hyperinfection syndrome thiabendazole 25 mg/kg twice daily for 15 days, in combination with an appropriate broad spectrum antibiotic, is of proven value, although the prognosis remains poor. Cambendazole, albendazole, ivermectin and cyclosporin A are all undergoing evaluation.

Prevention and control

Control measures are the same as for hookworm.

TRICHINOSIS

Aetiology and epidemiology

Trichinosis (trichiniasis) is caused by *Trichinella spiralis* and is cosmopolitan in man among pork-eating races. It is an important infection in areas of Europe and the USA, in sub-Saharan Africa and also in the Arctic. Two hosts are required for the parasite to be maintained, and each host is infected with both the adult and all the larval forms of the parasite. Man acquires the infection through the ingestion of infected meat, including pigs, horse and bear, containing encysted larvae.

The adult worms are present in the host small intestine. The female liberates larvae which penetrate the bowel wall and travel by both blood and lymph to muscle where they form cysts 1 mm in diameter. When meat or flesh is eaten raw or undercooked, the cyst wall is digested in the stomach and larvae escape into the duodenum, invade the mucosa and develop into short-lived adult parasites.

Domestic pigs provide a source of human infection. Pigs become infected by eating rats or offal in raw garbage or by nibbling at each other! In Africa the maintenance hosts of *Trichinella* are carrion feeding or cannibalistic wild carnivores, but human infections are almost always acquired by eating bushpigs or warthogs, which are secondary hosts. In the Arctic infection is acquired from polar bears and the walrus.

Clinical features

Light infections are often asymptomatic. In symptomatic cases symptoms are related to the parasitic invasion of the intestine, the migration of the larvae, and the encystment of larvae in muscle. About 7 days after eating infected meat the first symptoms may appear due to larval penetration of the bowel. There is an acute febrile illness with diarrhoea, abdominal pains and vomiting.

During the migratory phase the features of disease are severe myalgia, periorbital oedema, conjunctival and subungal haemorrhages and urticarial rashes. Possible complications include meningoencephalitis, myocarditis, pericardial effusion and Gram-negative bacterial septicaemia.

Diagnosis

Trichinosis is associated with a high eosinophilia, marked elevation of serum CPK, and ELISA or IFAT serology is positive. The presence of larvae within a muscle biopsy will confirm the diagnosis.

The differential diagnosis includes Katayama fever in schistosomiasis, disseminated strongyloidiasis, toxocariasis and poisoning by L-tryptophan or 'Spanish toxic oil'.

Treatment

Treatment is directed against the larvae and the immune response they invoke. Mebendazole 20 mg/kg 6 hourly for two weeks may be larvicidal. Albendazole may prove to be a superior treatment. In the severe acute phase of disease prednisolone may be used judiciously to control the inflammatory response elicited by the disseminated larvae.

Prevention and control

The larvae are killed by thorough cooking of meat and by irradiation. Infected carcasses can be recognized by means of trichinoscopy and rejected.

The larvae are also killed by freezing at $-15\,°C$ for 3 weeks, or sooner at lower temperatures.

Better animal husbandry with feeding of only cooked swill to pigs destined to provide pork meat will also prevent transmission of trichinosis.

TRICHURIASIS

Aetiology and epidemiology

The whipworm *Trichuris trichiura* has a worldwide distribution. The adult worms are 2–5 cm long, the thinner anterior half of the body being normally buried in the mucosa of the colon, caecum or rectum of the human host. Although they may cause haemorrhage at their site of attachment, they feed on tissue juices and not on blood. Mature female worms produce several thousand eggs per day which escape in the stool. After 2 weeks development in warm soil the eggs are embryonated and infective. Embryonated eggs ingested by man on contaminated fruits and vegetables hatch in the small intestine where they undergo development before proceeding to the large intestine, where they attach to the mucosa and become adult. The heaviest infections are in children who swallow most soil.

Clinical features

The majority of infections are light and asymptomatic. In severe infections there may be a dysentery-like illness with passage of blood and mucus in the stool. Haemorrhagic ulceration of the colonic mucosa occurs and may give rise to perforation and peritonitis. Rectal prolapse occurs not uncommonly in children and heavy infections may be associated with poor nutrition and growth retardation. *Trichuris* is commonly found in association with other bowel parasitic infections.

Diagnosis

Worms may be seen at proctoscopy. Eggs are found in the stool, measure 50 μm by 30 μm and are barrel-shaped and bile stained.

Treatment

Mebendazole and albendazole are both effective treatments.

Prevention and control

Prevention and control is the same as that for *Ascaris* – avoidance of soil contamination and mass chemotherapy initiatives.

VISCERAL LARVA MIGRANS

Many helminthic diseases could be regarded as causing 'visceral larva migrans' (cysticercosis, hydatidosis, strongyloidiasis, ancylostomiasis, filariasis) but the term is normally reserved for the pathology caused by the allergic reaction to larvae of *Toxocara canis* and *T. catis*, especially in children, as a result of the ingestion of soil contaminated with incubated embryonated eggs from dog or cat faeces, the hosts of the adult worms.

Infection in man may be inapparent or cause mild eosinophilia only, but can produce a severe illness with fever, hepatomegaly, lung infiltrates with wheezing and cough, and epilepsy. Within the eye it can induce a granulomatous eosinophilic endophthalmitis which may clinically resemble a retinoblastoma.

A reliable ELISA test is available for diagnosis. Symptomatic toxocariasis should be treated with albendazole or thiabendazole. Diethylcarbamazine has also been used.

Prevention depends on the regular deworming of domestic dogs and limiting environmental contamination with dog faeces.

10
Tapeworms (Cestodes)

Tapeworms belong to the phylum *Platyhelminthes* and the class *Cestoidea*. Platyhelminths are worms that are dorso-ventrally flattened. Two classes of this phylum contain parasites of medical importance to man; the *Cestoidea* or tapeworms and the *Trematoda* or flukes.

Tapeworms are parasites of the mammalian intestine. They have a head or scolex and a body made up of segments or proglottides. They are hermaphroditic, each segment containing both testes and ovary. The most important cestodes with respect to their clinical and public health importance belong to the family *Taeniidae* and include *Taenia saginata*, *T. solium*, *Echinococcus granulosus* and *E. multilocularis*. These adult tapeworms occur in the small intestine of their primary mammalian host; the secondary mammalian host is infected by ingesting eggs from faecal contamination of the primary host leading to the development of parasite larvae in the tissues.

TAENIA SAGINATA

Aetiology and epidemiology

Taenia saginata, the beef tapeworm, occurs in its adult form in the small intestine of man. The larval form, or cysticercus, is found in cattle, the secondary host. *Taenia saginata* has a worldwide distribution but is particularly frequent wherever beef is eaten raw or insufficiently cooked and where poor sanitation permits access of cattle to human faecal contamination.

The adult worm, usually occurring singly in man's small intestine, may grow up to a length of 10 m and consist of up to 2000 proglottides. The more mature posterior proglottides produce eggs in the uterus and eventually the distal gravid proglottides, each containing up to 100 000 eggs, are detached and pass down the intestine. The gravid proglottis migrates through the anus and eggs are released into the environment. The eggs, each of which contains a hexacanth embryo, may survive from days to months, depending upon environmental conditions. They depend for their further development on being ingested by a suitable cattle host. On ingestion by the secondary host the embryo is liberated, burrows through the intestinal wall and is carried by the circulation to muscle tissue, particularly the masseters, the tongue and the diaphragm, where it develops into a fluid filled cyst about 1×0.5 cm in size, a small invagination of which develops into a small head resembling that of the adult tapeworm.

This stage is known as a cysticercus, and meat consisting of flesh containing cysticerci is referred to as 'measly'. If man eats the raw or undercooked measly meat the wall of the cyst is digested and the scolex is liberated in the small intestine where it attaches itself to the wall by suckers and grows into adulthood.

Clinical features

Most tapeworm infections are asymptomatic and the adult worm may remain in the bowel for up to 30 years and produce no symptoms. The commonest clinical presentation is when the patient is aware of the discharge of gravid segments through the anus or of a crawling sensation in the perianal region. There is no evidence of malabsorption and only occasionally is there any significant loss of appetite sufficient to cause weight loss.

Diagnosis

The diagnosis is made by finding the gravid segments in a faecal sample. In *T. saginata* the uterus bears 18 to 30 compound branches on each side as counted from where they arise from the main uterine body, thus differentiating it from *T. solium* which has 8 to 12 uterine branches. These can be identified in a fresh specimen with the aid of a hand lens but identification is often made easier by utilizing staining techniques.

The eggs of *T. saginata* are spherical and brown in colour measuring some 30–40 μm in diameter with a thick radially striated wall. The eggs are indistinguishable from those of *T. solium*. They may be found in stool but are generally not released from the gravid segment until it has escaped through the anus.

Treatment

Treatment will be discussed in the section on *T. solium*, below.

Prevention and control

Measures for the prevention and control of *T. saginata* include:

1. improvements in health education and sanitation to prevent contamination of soil, water, pasture and animal feed with human faeces;
2. inspection of meat will detect many infected carcasses which should be condemned or suitably processed;
3. adequate cooking of beef will destroy cysticerci which are susceptible to temperatures in excess of 56 °C;
4. freezing beef to a temperature below −5 °C for >4 days kills cysticerci.

TAENIA SOLIUM

Aetiology and epidemiology

Man is the definitive host of the adult *T. solium* and the pig is the usual secondary host. *T. solium* has a cosmopolitan distribution, being most common wherever pork is eaten raw. Large series of cases attest to its frequency in Eastern Europe, China, India, Mexico, South American and South Africa.

The adult tapeworm has a length of 2–3 m with up to 1000 proglottides. The life cycle is similar to that of *T. saginata*. Eggs passed out with faeces are ingested by pigs and the liberated embryo develops in the porcine flesh to form a cysticercus some 0.5 × 1 cm in size. However in *T. solium*, unlike *T. saginata*, the eggs are also infective to man and cysticercosis may develop in man if he ingests faecal contaminated substances containing ova. Auto-infection may occur when a person infected with an adult tapeworm contaminates his or her hands and ingests tapeworm eggs. The long-held belief that regurgitation of tapeworm segments in the stomach as a result of vomiting with resultant release of embryonated eggs in the stomach may lead to the development of cysticercosis has never been verified. In man hexacanth embryos which hatch in the small intestine burrow into venules and are carried to distant sites, lodging most commonly in the brain and meninges, but also in muscle, eyes and other organs where they develop into mature larvae and encyst.

Clinical features

The clinical features of the adult *T. solium* are similar to those of *T. saginata*. When cysticerci develop in man symptoms are mainly due to invasion of the central nervous system. The clinical manifestations of cerebral cysticercosis are varied depending on the number of larvae, their location and the host response. Clinical presentation includes fits, focal deficits, increased intracranial pressure due to communicating and non-communicating hydrocephalus, and meningitis. Focal Jacksonian fits or generalized seizures occur in up to 92% of patients. In children who are more likely to ingest larger quantities of ova and hence have a greater parasitaemia, a clinical picture resembling acute encephalitis may be the initial presentation. A particularly severe and aggressive form of disease is found when groups of cysticerci arborize into extensive grape-like clusters around the basal cisterns with hydrocephalus and dementia as the outcome.

Diagnosis

Diagnosis of the adult worm is by the identification of gravid segments in a faecal sample. The uterus of *T. solium* differs from that of *T. saginata* in having 8 to 12 compound branches on each side of the uterine body. The eggs of *T. solium* and *T. saginata* are identical.

Computerized tomographic scanning (CT) and magnetic resonance (MR) imaging are useful in the diagnosis of cerebral cysticercosis and several patterns have been described. Parenchymal lesions are most common. Small (2–6 mm) round or oval calcifications represent dead calcified cysticerci. Calcified lesions show no perifocal oedema and no enhancement in post-contrast studies. Cysticerci in the form of cysts can be demonstrated and range in size from 0.5–3.0 cm and are of low attenuation on CT scans. The resolution with MR scans may permit the visualization of larval protoscolices within the cyst. These cysts may be associated with perifocal oedema and ring enhancement after administration of contrast material. In adults such lesions are usually few in number and when associated with seizures perifocal oedema is invariably noted. It is likely that there is little if any reaction of the brain to the cysticerci prior to their death and the living cysticercus may be isodense on CT scanning. Ring enhancement has been noted to develop after therapy with praziquantel, a larvicidal drug, suggesting this is a manifestation of an inflammatory response to the dying larva. It would appear that the death of the larva provokes an inflammatory reaction with perifocal cerebral oedema and that this precipitates neurological symptoms, especially focal epileptiform seizures.

In developing countries, investigation of patients with neurological symptoms is limited by economic factors and special radiological studies are often available only to privileged members of the population.

Several serological tests have been developed for detection of antibodies as a diagnostic procedure with varying degrees of success in the diagnosis of human cysticercosis. Most are beset by the problems of antigen specificity and sensitivity especially in areas where other cestode infections are endemic. Some ELISA tests have shown promise, but to date an enzyme-linked immunotransfer blot (EITB) assay has provided the most precise method of diagnosing cysticercosis in neurological patients. Until sophisticated radiological and serological investigations are more readily available in the developing world the diagnosis of cysticercosis will remain difficult. Presumptive diagnosis often rests on a history of exposure in an endemic area and the finding of subcutaneous or intramuscular nodules on careful palpation of the whole body. Excision and histological examination of superficial nodules will confirm or otherwise the diagnosis of cysticercosis but will not prove causation of neurological symptoms.

Differential diagnosis

Neurocysticercosis may manifest itself in multifarious ways and encompass a wide number of differential diagnoses. In many areas of the world tuberculosis occurs where cysticercosis is endemic. Confusion has arisen in the interpretation of solitary ring enhancing lesions on CT scanning in this situation as both cerebral cysticercosis and cerebral tuberculomas may give rise to a similar CT appearance. A single ring enhancing lesion has been reported in 26% of Indian patients with seizures and these lesions are commonly managed as tuberculomas. In one such series however, excision biopsy demonstrated the presence of cysticerci in 12 of 15 consecutive patients with no tuberculomas being recorded. Care must be taken in making this difficult differential diagnosis.

The average interval from initial infection with cysticercosis to onset of cerebral symptoms is approximately 5 years, with a range of a few months to 30 years. A diagnosis of cerebral cysticercosis should therefore be considered in any patient presenting with epileptiform seizures who has spent time in an area where cysticercosis is known to be endemic.

Treatment

The drug of choice for the treatment of both *T. solium* and *T. saginata* adult tapeworms is praziquantel in a single dose of 10 mg/kg. As internal auto-infection with *T. solium* has not been demonstrated, purging of the patient after treatment is not required. Niclosamide (Yomesan) is an alternative treatment given as chewable tablets in two doses of 1 g taken at hourly intervals.

Praziquantel was first reported as a treatment for cysticercosis in pigs in 1978 and in man in 1980. Treatment with praziquantel has been demonstrated to reduce the number and size of cysticercal cysts. The dramatic host reaction which can develop around the cysts during treatment can lead to the development of increased symptoms and severe intracranial hypertension. Dexamethasone should be used in conjunction with praziquantel to reduce cerebral oedema and its sequelae. Treatment with praziquantel can lead to the complete resolution on CT scanning of the ring enhancing lesion and surrounding oedema. Residual areas of calcification may appear at the site of the lesion. Although spontaneous resolution of lesions has been observed in the absence of specific treatment the rationale for treatment in patients who on CT scans appear to have few cerebral cysticerci is to kill any live cysticerci which may have escaped detection (often being isodense on CT), under the control of the inflammatory suppressant action of dexamethasone. A suggested treatment regimen is praziquantel 50 mg/kg daily in three divided doses for 15 days. Dexamethasone 2 mg three times a day should be started 2 days prior to praziquantel treatment, the dosage being tapered off during therapy. Both albendazole and flubendazole have been used successfully in the treatment of cerebral cysticercosis but have not yet been fully evaluated.

Surgery has a role in the management of patients with intraventricular cysts and hydrocephalus where the results of chemotherapy are usually disappointing.

Prevention and control

Man is the sole definitive host of *T. solium* and therefore health education is of paramount importance. Indiscriminate human defaecation must be strongly discouraged. Identification and immediate treatment of persons harbouring adult *T. solium* must be encouraged.

Husbandry practices must be improved to prevent pigs access to human faecally contaminated foodstuffs.

The source of human infection with *T. solium* is infected pork and risk can be minimized by thorough meat inspection, adequate cooking, or killing of cysticerci by freezing as described for *T. saginata*.

HYDATID DISEASE

Hydatid disease is caused by the cestode tapeworm *Echinococcus* which belongs to the phylum *Platyhelminthes*, order *Cyclophyllidea* and family *Taeniidae*. Hydatid disease in man is caused by the larval stage of the canine tapeworm *Echinococcus granulosus*, which more usually has sheep or other herbivores as its intermediate host, and less commonly by *E. multilocularis*, which has its normal intermediate stage in rodents.

ECHINOCOCCUS GRANULOSUS

Aetiology and epidemiology

The worldwide occurrence of the intermediate hosts (sheep, cattle, etc.) and of dog, the definitive host, has led to a cosmopolitan distribution of *E. granulosus* hydatid disease. The areas where it is most commonly found are within the cattle and sheep rearing countries of Australia, New Zealand, Argentina, the Middle East, South Africa and many parts of Europe. The Turkana, a pastoral tribe living in the desert region of north western Kenya, seem to have one of the highest incidences of human hydatid disease in the world due to close association between the members of their tribe and their dogs. Human cases are seen in the UK in emigrants from endemic regions and also indigenous cases from farming regions such as Powys in Wales, where there is a recorded incidence of up to one new case per 700 population per annum.

Echinococcus granulosus is found in the adult form attached to the mucosa of the small intestine of both wild and domestic canines. The worm is very small, ranging from 2–9 mm in length with a maximum breadth of 500 μm. It is composed of a head and three segments, the distal segment being somewhat longer than the rest of the worm. The first segment contains no reproductive organs, the second is mature, and the third is gravid. Eggs in the faeces of the dog host are infective to man, and to herbivorous domestic and wild animal hosts. They are indistinguishable from the *Taenia* eggs previously described. Once ingested the larval form is liberated from the egg and penetrates the intestinal mucosa to invade practically every organ in the body, but is most commonly found in the liver and lungs. The larva develops into a hydatid cyst which is made up of a fibrous layer of host origin surrounding the cyst and an inner germinal layer from which brood capsules and daughter cysts arise. Larval scolices arise from the wall of the brood capsule, which evaginates to provide a protective cup. When the cyst is eaten by the definitive canine host the scolex evaginates and attaches to the intestinal mucosa where it develops into an adult tapeworm.

Canines are infected by eating the cysts in dead herbivores or in their discarded offal and convey the infection to man by close contact and the fouling of the environment.

Clinical features

Hydatid cysts present as mass lesions either as an incidental finding on radiological investigation of non-related symptoms or because of symptoms or signs secondary to progressive expansion of the cyst. Liver and lung involvement are most commonly found.

Liver hydatids commonly present as an abdominal mass. Distension of the liver capsule may cause discomfort or pain. Cysts may be so large as to distort and obstruct the portal vessels giving rise to portal hypertension. Jaundice may result from pressure on the bile ducts and cholangitis from rupture into the biliary tree. Lung lesions are often found on routine radiological examination. Shortness of breath and chest pain may be present if the cyst is large and the cyst may give rise to bronchial obstruction and collapse of the lobe. Haemoptysis may follow the ulceration of a bronchus and, following the rupture of a cyst into the bronchial tree, the patient may expectorate daughter cysts and watery fluid.

Respiratory distress may ensue as a result of cyst fluid aspiration and may be associated with urticaria or anaphylactic shock. The clinical picture of cerebral enchinococcosis is similar to other conditions causing space occupying lesions and a slowly increased intracranial pressure.

Renal hydatid cysts may present with haematuria and require differentiation from a hypernephroma. Cysts in bone can lead to spontaneous pathological fractures and vertebral compression fractures.

Diagnosis

The absence of an appropriate geographical history and no contact with dogs makes the diagnosis unlikely.

Plain radiography is the most useful method in the diagnosis of pulmonary cysts. The cyst is demonstrated as a rounded, well-defined, uniformly dense lesion. If the cyst dies its wall may calcify. Rupture of the cyst may give rise to the appearance of a fluid level within the cyst. Ultrasound examination is useful particularly when applied to the liver and other abdominal viscera, and computerized tomography is the imaging investigation of choice for intracerebral lesions. Cerebral cysts do not enhance nor do they give rise to perifocal oedema.

Immunodiagnosis has a role in identifying hydatid disease. The latex agglutination test is a good screening test with high specificity. The complement fixation test (CFT) is positive in up to 80% of patients. Immunoelectrophoresis is the most specific test in general use and along with the CFT is used to confirm the diagnosis.

An eosinophilia is present in up to 30% of cases, but is non-specific.

Treatment

Surgery has been the main line of management and a cyst giving rise to symptoms is preferably removed. This is often technically demanding and may involve partial or complete removal of the organ involved. Rupture of a cyst during removal can lead to spillage of daughter cysts and protoscolices, resulting in dissemination of the hydatid disease. A more immediate complication of spillage of cyst contents is the development of anaphylactic shock. The use of scolicidal agents, such as 0.1% cetrimide solution, is well established in the operative management of hydatid cysts for the packing of the operative field and for injection into the cysts themselves to minimize the risk of dissemination if spillage should occur.

Chemotherapy is now able to make a contribution to management. Mebendazole was the first drug demonstrated to be active against hydatid disease but is relatively insoluble and poorly absorbed and only produced limited success when given in large and potentially toxic doses. More recently albendazole has been demonstrated to be better absorbed, to penetrate cysts and to be protoscolicidal. Evidence currently available suggests that albendazole may be used as a prophylactic measure, as an adjunct to surgery, and may achieve some therapeutic success when given in inoperable cases. The current recommended dosage regimen is albendazole 800 mg daily in cycles of 28 days with 14 day intervals between cycles, with a mean of 2.5 cycles (range 1–12).

Praziquantel, used successfully to treat adult worms, has no effect on mature cysts. It is however active against protoscolices and may be given in the perioperative period to reduce the risk of accidental dissemination.

Prevention and control

Infection in dogs can be prevented by curbing the indiscriminate disposal of offal and the controlled slaughter of herbivorous animal stock in authorized areas free from dogs. Dogs at risk by virtue of their occupational exposure to animals should be periodically treated with praziquantel. Infection in man can be prevented by educating those in endemic areas to control environmental contamination by dog faeces and to minimize their close contact with dogs.

ECHINOCOCCUS MULTILOCULARIS

Aetiology and epidemiology

The distribution of *Echinococcus multilocularis* is mainly arctic and alpine but has been reported in India and Iraq. The adult tapeworm is found in the intestine of canids and the cyst in the live of small rodents. Man is infected by ingesting eggs on raw fruit and vegetables that have been contaminated by the faeces of infected canids.

Clinical features

As its name implies, cysts of *E. multilocularis* are multilocular. The cysts are in fact often more solid that cystic, giving rise to an irregular alveolar or honeycombed structure which tends to be invasive and to metastasize to other organs. The primary lesion, which often does not present until many years after infection, is invariably hepatic and may present with pain and hepatomegaly, as portal hypertension or with jaundice. Metastases to the brain and lungs are not infrequent.

Diagnosis

Ultrasound or computerized tomography of the liver will demonstrate a diffuse, partially cystic mass which must be differentiated from a hepatoma. Serodiagnosis is usually performed using purified *E. multilocularis* antigen in an indirect haemagglutination test.

Treatment

Because of the invasive and metastatic nature of the disease complete surgical removal and cure is rarely achievable. Albendazole may prove useful in limiting the spread of disease.

Prevention and control

Treatment of dogs with praziquantel and food hygiene are the mainstays of prevention.

11
Filariasis and Onchocerciasis

INTRODUCTION

The nematode worms which are tissue parasites of man are listed in Table 11.1. All except *Dracunculus medinensis* are transmitted by arthropod vectors in the form of filarial larvae, and all exist as slowly-maturing male and female adults living in tissues in lymphatics and lymph nodes. They cause human disease only on repeated exposure; the pathology results from tissue and allergic reactions to migrating larvae and adult worms.

LYMPHATIC FILARIASIS

Lymphatic filariasis is caused by *Wuchereria bancrofti*, *Brugia malayi* and *Brugia timori*. The adult worms (male 40×0.1 mm, female 100×0.3 mm) live in lymph nodes and vessels. The female releases larval microfilariae which are disseminated into the blood. If ingested by mosquitoes the microfilariae develop into infective larvae which are transmitted through the saliva of the female mosquito.

Nocturnally periodic strains of *W. bancrofti* are transmitted in urban areas of the tropics by peridomestic *Culex*, e.g. *quinquefasciatus* and in the rural tropics by *Anopheles* species. A non-periodic strain, *W. bancrofti*, in Polynesia has *Aedes* species as its vector. Bancroftian filariasis has its reservoir of infection only in man.

Brugia malayi has a nocturnally periodic strain only found in man which is transmitted by anopheline and other mosquitoes in swamps and paddy fields, and a semi-periodic strain which has a reservoir in felines and monkeys which is transmitted in swamps and forests by *Mansonia spp.*

Brugia timori is a human parasite transmitted by anophelines.

Table 11.1 Nematode tissue parasites

Parasite	Distribution	Vector	Main Pathology
Wuchereria bancrofti			
i) nocturnally periodic	Tropical Africa	Urban-*Culex* mosq	Lymphatic
	S. America	Rural-*Aphopheles* mosq	
	India		
	S.E. Asia		
	China		
ii) non-periodic	Polynesia	*Aedes* mosq	
Brugia malayi			
i) nocturnally periodic	S.E. Asia	*Anopheles* mosq	Lymphatic
		Mansonia mosq	
		Aedes mosq	
ii) semi-periodic	SE Asia	*Mansonia* mosq	
Brugia timori (nocturnally periodic)	Indonesia (Timor & Flores)	*Anopheles* mosq	Lymphatic
Onchocerca volvulus	Africa	*Simulium*	Skin, eye
	C. and S. America		
Loa loa	W. Africa	*Chrysops*	Skin
Mansonella perstans	Africa	*Culicoides*	Serosa
	S. America		
Mansonella streptocerca	Africa	*Culicoides*	Skin
Mansonella ozzardi	C. and S. America	*Culicoides*	Skin
Dracunculus medinensis	Africa	*Cyclops* (ingested)	Skin
	India		
	Pakistan		

The pathology of filarial infection (as with some other metazoan parasites, e.g. schistosomes) is conditioned by a symbiotic relationship between the host and the adult worms and microfilariae in which the natural immune responses of the host are 'down-regulated' to produce a state of balanced immune tolerance. The IgE response is modulated by 'blocking' IgG antibodies. When this balance is upset, by mechanisms which are not well understood, allergic reactions to the parasite cause tissue damage and systemic symptoms. Repeated infection leads to chronic damage to lymphatic vessels and lymph nodes; fibrosis and narrowing result in chronic lymphoedema ('elephantiasis'), especially in dependent areas such as the legs and scrotum. Early in the history of the infection, and intermittently thereafter, patients suffer episodes of fever, with eosinophilia, lymphangitis, lymphandenitis and epididymo-orchitis. Most of the pathology in lymphatic filariasis results from the host response to adult worms; microfilariae, although circulating in decreasing numbers as immune tolerance develops, do not cause disease, except in a small number of individuals on a genetic basis (e.g. certain Indian races) who respond with tropical pulmonary eosinophilia syndrome (TPE), in which a marked eosinophilic reaction occurs in the lungs, leading to fibrotic damage, but without microfilaraemia.

The clinical presentation of filarial infection is very variable; residents of endemic areas may have:

1. microfilaraemia without symptoms;
2. episodes of fever, lymphadenitis and retrograde lymphangitis for a few days, several times a year, with transient lymphoedema. Pyogenic abscesses may occur as a complication, and epididymo-orchitis is seen in young males, who may develop a serous or chylous hydrocoele;
3. after many years of exposure and recurrent lymphatic damage, progressive permanent lymphoedema, skin nodules and thickening and chyluria due to involvement of retroperitoneal tissues;
4. tropical pulmonary eosinophilia (TPE), in those susceptible, who develop cough with wheezing, dyspnoea and pulmonary fibrosis.

Non-immune expatriates are likely to suffer attacks of lymphangitis, lymphadenitis, hydrocoele, urticaria, angio-oedema and eosinophilia, without fever or microfilaraemia, which usually subside naturally without causing chronic disease if re-exposure does not occur.

Filarial elephantiasis should be distinguished from clinically similar podoconiosis in Africa and Central and South America, in which leg lymphatics are damaged by skin penetration of dust from red laterite volcanic clays containing iron and silicates.

The diagnosis of filariasis depends on the demonstration of microfilariae in blood, hydrocoele fluid or chylous urine.

Periodic parasites are found optimally in blood taken between 22.00 and 04.00 hours in wet smear or films stained with Giemsa; sub-periodic parasites may be found at any time, especially about 16.00 hours. Micropore filtration methods can be used to concentrate the fluid being examined. If microfilaraemia is absent, the diagnosis may be suspected from a high blood eosinophilia with a markedly raised serum IgE level, and confirmed by specific antifilaria IgG and IgE antibodies by CFT, IFAT or ELISA methods.

Filariasis may be treated with:

1. diethyl carbamazine (DEC), a piperazine derivative, which is an effective microfilaricide but has much less effect on adult worms. The standard oral dose is 6 mg/kg per day for 12 days, but 2 mg/kg may be given weekly over a longer period. In higher doses, symptoms produced by the allergic reaction to rapidly killed microfilariae include fever, headaches, chills and dizziness, especially in Brugia infections. This may be prevented by starting with a lower dose and increasing gradually, and may require additional treatment with antihistamines or corticosteroids;
2. ivermectin (IVM) is a potent microfilaricide in a single dose, with no effect on adult worms. A single intramuscular dose of 200–400 μg/kg is given.

In endemic areas long-term cure does not occur with these regimens, since the adult worms survive, but microfilaraemia can be suppressed by further doses. Established elephantiasis is unlikely to respond to medication; elastic stockings and scrotal supports may be helpful. Surgical drainage of hydrocoeles is useful, but heroic lymphatic surgery is impractical.

Control of filariasis is based on:

1. reduction of mosquito vector populations, which is only likely to be practical for urban and peridomestic species, by using insecticides;

2. mass chemotherapy of a population with a high incidence, e.g. annual treatment with DEC or IVM.

Chemoprophylaxis of non-immunes at special risk could be achieved with DEC (which is used in dogs for canine filariasis) or ivermectin, but this has not been widely used.

LOIASIS

The nematode worm *Loa loa*, whose adult forms migrate in subcutaneous tissues, is transmitted by the day-biting tabanid horse and deer fly *Chrysops dimidiata* in its microfilarial larval form, which circulates in the blood with a periodicity peaking at about 12.00 hours. The usual clinical presentation is with allergic ('Calabar') swellings, mainly on the limbs, which are painful and show non-pitting oedema, extend up to 10 cm in diameter, and last for 1 to 3 days. In residents of endemic areas, considerable microfilaraemia may be present with few symptoms; in expatriates, Calabar swellings and high eosinophilia are characteristic, and microfilariae may be scanty or absent in the blood.

A number of complications are possible:
1. encephalopathy in reaction to migrating microfilariae;
2. immune-complex nephrophathy;
3. cardiomyopathy or endomyocardial fibrosis (mediated by eosinophils);
4. the adult worms may migrate across the conjunctiva; this is visible and alarming to the patient but does not damage the eye permanently;
5. arthritis reactive to migration of adult worms in or near the synovium.

Loiasis is diagnosed by demonstrating microfilariae in stained day-time blood films. If these are absent, the history, together with eosinophilia and a positive serological test (CFT), will justify treatment.

Loiasis is treated with oral diethylcarbamazine (DEC) 8–10 mg/kg daily for 2 to 3 weeks: if microfilaraemia is high, generalized allergic reactions to treatment may occur and require the addition of antihistamines or corticosteroids. Alternatively a single intramuscular or oral dose of ivermectin 200–400 µg/kg can be given with less risk of allergic reactions. Accessible adult worms can be removed surgically.

Loiasis is an exclusively human disease which occurs only in the rain forests of West and Central Africa, and also in southern Sudan. Prevention in local populations can be assisted by the clearing of forests near villages; mass chemotherapy has not been attempted. Expatriates can be protected by weekly DEC 300 mg, if they are at special risk.

MANSONELLA PERSTANS (DIPETALONEMA PERSTANS)

The adults of this worm live in the peritoneal, pleural and pericardial cavities, mesentery and retroperitoneal tissues, but elicit remarkably little host response in many of those infected. There is a non-periodic microfilaraemia and the vector is the *Culicoides* midge. There is no animal reservoir. Some individuals suffer from 'Calabar'-like swelling, arthritis, angio-oedema and pericarditis, and occasional cases of retroperitoneal fibrosis with hydronephosis and chyluria occur. Diagnosis is by demonstration of microfilaraemia and treatment with DEC 6 mg/kg daily for 10–20 days. The infection occurs widely in sub-Saharan Africa.

MANSONELLA STREPTOCERCA

The subcutaneous adult worms of this parasite produce microfilariae which also inhabit subcutaneous tissues and which must be distinguished from those of *Onchocerca volvulus* in skin snip preparations by their hooked tail which contains nuclei to the tip. Many of those infected have no symptoms but the skin damage in some – papules, excoriation, hypopigmentation – should be distinguished from that in onchocerciasis and leprosy. Treatment if necessary is with DEC; the vector is the *Culicoides* midge, and the parasite is found in sub-Saharan Africa. Chimpanzees form an animal reservoir of infection.

ONCHOCERCIASIS

Onchocerca volvulus is an important cause of blindness and skin damage which infects 18–20 million people worldwide, mainly in sub-Saharan Africa, but also in Yemen, Mexico and northern South America. The adult worms live in subcutaneous tissues; pathological changes result mainly from the allergic response to microfilarial larvae in the skin, lymph nodes and eyes. The adults are very long thin worms (female 25–70 cm × 0.3 mm, male

3–6 cm × 0.15 mm) which are found coiled up in large numbers in subcutaneous nodules within a fibrous capsule. Microfilariae in the skin are transmitted from man to man by *Simulium* species of biting black flies (*S. damnosum*, *S. naevi*, etc.), the females of which lay their eggs for preference in vegetation attached to rocks or crabs at the edge of fast flowing well-oxygenated rivers. There is no animal reservoir of infection.

Microfilariae in the skin elicit an allergic response which causes hyperkeratosis, lymphatic damage, loss of elastic fibres and fibrosis and atrophy, and in the eye results in a heavy infiltrate of plasma cells and eosinophils which cause sclerosing keratitis, anterior uveitis, choroido-retinitis and finally optic atrophy.

The earliest clinical symptoms in the skin are of localized itching, with or without visible papule formation, in the buttocks and shoulders. Subsequently skin irritation spreads more widely, leading to generalized itching, with redness, swelling, papules, and excoriation from scratching. Over some months the skin becomes wrinkled, atrophic and patchily depigmented. Inguino-femoral adenopathy, with loose overlying skin, produces the 'hanging groin' appearance typical of the disease. Nodules containing adult worms are found in the skin of the pelvic region, chest wall and head. Involvement of the eye may present initially as an acutely red eye with keratitis, photophobia and watering; this will be followed by sclerosing keratitis, progressing from the limbus inwards, with opacification of the cornea, irregularity of the pupil, glaucoma and blindness as a result of damage to the cornea, choroid, retina and optic nerve.

Diagnosis of onchocerciasis is clinical in the first instance by examination of the subject for nodules, skin and eye changes. Final proof rests on the demonstration of microfilariae, emerging after incubation in isotonic saline for a few hours, in a small snip of skin or punch biopsy. A standard snipping technique allows this method also to produce a quantitative assessment of the infection. Onchocercal microfilariae should be distinguished from those of *Mansonella streptocerca* (see above). Excision biopsy of subcutaneous nodules shows existence of adult *Onchocerca* worms.

The diagnosis in expatriates who have had a relatively small exposure may be difficult, in that skin snips may show no microfilariae. Eosinophilia, with a positive serological test and a history of exposure, will suggest the diagnosis.

Onchocerciasis is treated with ivermectin in a single oral (fasting) dose of 150–200 µg/kg. An allergic (Mazzotti) reaction to the killed microfilariae, with skin oedema, increased itching and a maculo-papular rash, is unusual in residents of endemic countries, but may occur in expatriates. Retreatment, at intervals of 6–12 months, of residents is necessary to suppress microfilaria production and to control transmission. The treatment does not affect the adult worms, which may live for many years. Previously onchocerciasis was treated with DEC 1 mg/kg twice daily for 2 to 3 weeks, starting with a low dose (e.g. 25 mg) and building up to the full dose over the first week, in an attempt to reduce the effects of the Mazzotti reaction, which manifested as lymphadenitis, fever, headache, nausea, vomiting, and aggravation of the eye pathology with redness, photophobia and reduced vision. This reaction is treated with corticosteroids, both systemically and topically in the eye, and aspirin or other non-steroidal anti-inflammatory drugs.

The only agent of proven efficacy in killing adult worms is suramin, but this is given intravenously and causes risks of serious toxicity. Surgical nodulectomy, especially in the head and neck region, to reduce the load of microfilariae reaching the eyes, is a useful adjunct in management.

The control of onchocerciasis depends on:

1. reduction of *Simulium* vector populations. This has been attempted on a large scale in West Africa by spraying the larvicide 'temephos' into rivers from helicopters; this is expensive and may induce resistance to the agent in the fly population, and is inappropriate in environments which are ecologically unsuitable (e.g. open farmland in the early wet season) but where transmission occurs;
2. mass chemotherapy of infected human populations using 6 or 12-monthly doses of ivermectin (see above);
3. education and management of populations so that infected areas are evacuated, new villages in cleared areas provided, and the people discouraged from using rivers where *Simulium* breeds for washing, drawing water or playing.

DRACONTIASIS

Dracontiasis is caused by the 'Guinea worm', *Dracunculus medinensis*, which is transmitted to man by the ingestion of water containing its larvae within a small freshwater crustacean – the water-flea *Cyclops*. Larvae penetrate the small intestine and mature in the peritoneal cavity; mating of male and female worms occurs and the male then dies. The gravid female worm (60–100 cm × 1.5–2 mm) migrates so that her tail lies within a skin blister, usually on the lower leg, which bursts to liberate larvae on exposure to water. This is an exclusively human parasite.

The usual clinical presentation is with a painful inflamed itching ulcer on the lower leg or foot, in which the tail of the worm may be visible, but the lesion can occur anywhere on the body surface, and the worms may migrate to the spinal cord, brain or heart with serious or lethal effects. The skin ulcer is often infected by bacteria, and may provide the portal of entry for tetanus spores. Adjacent joints may become inflamed, and later ankylosed. Fever and systemic allergic symptoms occur unusually.

The diagnosis is usually clinical; differentiation should be made from *Loa loa*, cutaneous larva migrans, Buruli ulcer, neuropathic ulceration in leprosy and mycetoma.

The most effective treatment is physical removal of the female worm (e.g. by carefully rolling it onto a stick) but this must await the emergence of the tail, which can be encouraged by immersion in water.

Niridazole and metronidazole have been used to reduce the inflammatory reaction but do not kill the worm. The ulcer should be cleaned, disinfected and dressed, and tetanus prophylaxis given.

The infection occurs in West Africa, especially in Benin, Ghana, Nigeria and Burkina Faso, and in India and Pakistan. Considerable progress has been made in controlling the disease by educating people in rural communities to boil or filter drinking water (e.g. through two layers of muslin), by the provision of protected water supplies (e.g. step wells) and by the introduction of 'tempehos' as a larvicide for *Cyclops* into pools, tanks and wells. WHO regards dracontiasis as a potentially eradicable disease.

12

Schistosomiasis and Human Fluke Infections

Trematode parasites of man and animals can be divided into two classes: schistosomes and hermaphrodite flukes. Hermaphrodite flukes have a mammalian definitive host, snails as a first intermediate host, and crustacea, fish or vegetation as second intermediate hosts. Flukes of the genera *Clonorchis*, *Opisthorchis* and *Fasciola* infect the biliary tract, *Fasciolopsis* the small intestine, and *Paragonimus* the bronchial tree of man.

SCHISTOSOMIASIS

Schistosomiasis ('bilharzia') is caused by three flukes or trematode flatworms whose adult forms inhabit the veins of abdominal viscera; the pathology which they cause results from the host immune response to the eggs they produce. Eggs excreted in human urine or faeces contaminating fresh water transform into motile larvae (miracidia) which then penetrate certain species of snail living in the water. After a period of development, actively motile cercarial larvae are released which attach to and penetrate human skin. They may die there if the host mounts an efficient immune response; if not, the cercariae modify their antigenic surface so as to be immunologically acceptable and pass in the bloodstream through the lungs to visceral veins, where adult flukes develop in copulating pairs, the female lying in a groove in the body of the male. *Schistosoma mansoni* adults inhabit the superior mesenteric veins, *S. haematobium* the veins of the urinary bladder, and *S. japonicum* the inferior mesenteric veins. *S. haematobium* females release terminally-spined ova into the urine, and *S. mansoni* laterally-spined ova, and *S. japonicum* ova with a lateral knob' into the intestinal lumen to complete the life cycles.

Cercarial penetration of the skin elicits an immediate allergic response which causes an itching maculo-papular rash ('cercarial dermatitis' or 'swimmer's itch'). This is prominent with S. mansoni, less so with S. haematobium and usually absent with S. japonicum.

The infection is then silent until the adult flukes have matured and started to release ova into the blood vessels. A generalized allergic illness known as 'Katayama syndrome' then occurs 2 to 10 weeks after the original invasion. This is characterized by fever, cough, hepatic and splenic enlargement, urticaria, eosinophilia, diarrhoea and, in severe cases, myocarditis and encephalopathy which may result in death. Established chronic infection causes disease through tissue immune response to ova which lead to granuloma formation, and fibrosis, of special importance in the liver and lungs. Ova disseminated to the brain and spinal cord may cause encephalopathy and transverse myelitis.

S. haematobium adults live in the veins of the urinary bladder, and start to produce eggs 4–9 weeks after cercarial invasion. Katayama fever is mild or absent; the earliest clinical symptom is haematuria, often at the end of micturition. Cystoscopy at this stage shows patchy inflammation and oedema with ulcers, nodules and pseudopapillomas, which biopsy shows to consist of granulomas surrounding each egg, deposited under the mucosal surface. Involvement of the ureteric orifices in this process may cause obstructive uropathy, but this often subsides without treatment. Subsequently fibrosis and calcification of the bladder wall occur, and secondary bacterial infection may be present.

Squamous carcinoma of the bladder is a possible complication of the chronic inflammation of the mucosa.

S. haematobium infection is diagnosed by the demonstration of ova in the sediment or microfiltrate of urine passed between 12.00 and 15.00 hours, in which red blood cells will usually also be seen. Ultrasound or intravenous urography are used to assess the effects on the bladder wall, uterus and kidneys, and cystoscopy with biopsy will show the characteristic appearances and histology. Eosinophilia is mild or absent. Treatment is with oral metriphonate 7.5–10 mg/kg in three fortnightly doses, or with a single oral dose of praziquantel 40 mg/kg. Metriphonate is an organophosphate and so should be used with caution in individuals exposed to related insecticides.

S. mansoni causes itching cercarial dermatitis, starting on the day of exposure and then subsiding. Katayama fever occurs 2 to 9 weeks later. Chronic infection results in inflammatory pseudopolyposis of the colon (especially the rectum and sigmoid colon), with an ulcerated granular mucosal surface, which causes intermittent bloody diarrhoea with abdominal pain. Ova carried in the portal veins to the liver elicit a periportal granulomatous response, followed by fibrosis, which results in firm smooth uncomfortable enlargement of the liver, splenomegaly, and portal hypertension complicated by ascites and oesophageal varices, but usually without jaundice or hepatic decompensation unless the patient also has chronic hepatitis B virus (HBV) infection or is an alcoholic. Porto-systemic shunting of blood allows ova to pass to the pulmonary veins, where the inflammatory and fibrotic response may lead to the development of pulmonary hypertension and 'cor pulmonale'.

Patients with chronic *S. mansoni* infection are particularly susceptible to recurrent fever due to blood infection with *Salmonella typhi* and *paratyphi*.

S. mansoni infection is diagnosed by the demonstration of ova in the stool, preferably in formol-ether concentrates. Confirmatory evidence can be provided by ultrasound examination of the liver to show periportal fibrosis, and biopsy of the rectal mucosa or liver which shows eosinophilic material in a fibrotic granuloma around ova (the Hoeppli reaction). A sensitive serum ELISA test can be used in early or mild infections. Treatment is with a single oral dose of praziquantel 40 mg/kg or with oral oxamniquine 20 (up to 60) mg/kg once. Patients with hepatic fibrosis may show improvement after treatment, but if bleeding from oesophageal varices occurs, endoscopic sclerosing injections and porto-systemic shunting surgery can be employed.

S. japonicum rarely causes cercarial dermatitis. The Katayama syndrome is serious and common, and typically occurs 5–8 weeks after invasion. Death may occur from acute encephalopathy or myocarditis. Chronic infection causes recurrent abdominal pain and bloody diarrhoea, with hepatic pulmonary and cardiac complications similar to those caused by *S. mansoni*. Chronic encephalopathy may cause epilepsy. The diagnosis is made by demonstration of ova in faecal concentrates. A serum ELISA test is available. Treatment is with oral praziquantel 50 mg/kg once or 20 mg/kg weekly for three doses.

S. haematobium disease occurs in sub-Saharan Africa from the Atlantic coast to Western Kenya, South-east Africa, Madagascar,

Mauritius, the Nile valley, Western Arabia and Iraq. Human patients are the only source of infection to the intermediate *Bulinus* snail hosts by the contamination of rivers, streams, canals, irrigated land and lakes by urine. *S. mansoni* occurs in sub-Saharan Africa, Sudan, Ethiopia, Arabia and the Nile delta, and Brazil and some Caribbean islands where infected human faeces contaminate fresh water containing *Biomphalaria* snails. *S. japonicum* occurs in Japan, the Yangtze valley of China, Cambodia, Thailand and peninsular Malaysia, mainly in rice-growing areas. In addition to the human source, which is important because faeces are commonly used as fertilizer, many animal species (domestic bovines, rodents) act as an additional reservoir of this infection. The snail host is *Onchomelania*.

Prevention and control of schistosomiasis depends on:

1. provision of safe water supplies and effective latrines, with education in the use of the latter;
2. health education to reduce human contact with infected freshwater sources, especially swimming;
3. correct management of irrigation schemes to avoid snail breeding;
4. mass chemotherapy of infected human populations; this has been particularly successful when targeted on school-age children who often have the highest burden of worms and eggs, and the most exposure. Praziquantel can be used for all species, metriphonate for *S. haematobium*, oxamniquine for *S. mansoni*;
5. reduction of snail populations by treating water with molluscicides (e.g. niclosamide) or by introducing molluscivorous fish or competitor molluscs which are not intermediate hosts;
6. development of vaccines employing certain polypeptide antigens present in the integument of the fluke.

LIVER FLUKE DISEASES OF MAN

Clonorchis sinensis, Opisthorchis felineus and *Opisthorchis viverrini* are the species which commonly infect man. *Clonorchis* is endemic in China, Japan, Korea, Taiwan and Vietnam. Reservoir hosts include domestic cats and dogs. *Opisthorchis felineus* is found in Eastern Europe, Russia and India as a widespread zoonosis, whilst *O. viverrini* is most common in Thailand, Cambodia and Laos with cats, dogs and fish-eating mammals as significant reservoirs.

Clonorchis sinensis

Aetiology and epidemiology

The adult *Clonorchis* inhabits the bile ducts of man and measures about 1 to 2 cm in length and 5 mm or less in breadth. The almost transparent body is stained browny-red with bile and possesses an oral sucker surrounding the mouth anteriorly and, a little behind it, a large ventral sucker. This hermaphrodite fluke produces flask-shaped operculated eggs, which measure about $30 \times 16\ \mu m$ and contain a ciliated larva or miracidium, which are passed with the bile into the intestine. Eggs are passed in the faeces which may then contaminate fresh water. For further development the egg containing a mature miracidium must be ingested by a suitable snail host. In the snail the miracidium develops into a sporocyst and then a redia before the mature redia bursts releasing cercariae into the surrounding water. When a cercaria comes into contact with a susceptible species of fish it penetrates between its scales and invades its flesh where it encysts. Man eating raw, pickled or undercooked fish ingests the cysts which are digested in the duodenum, releasing metacercariae which then migrate up the bile duct where they develop into adult flukes.

It is estimated that 19 million persons in the Far East are infected with *C. sinensis*.

Clinical features

Symptoms of clonorchiasis are thought to be related to the fluke burden. Persons harbouring fewer than 100 flukes are usually asymptomatic. Those with burdens of 100 to fewer than 1000 flukes often have non-specific symptoms, such as anorexia, nausea, epigastric pain and diarrhoea. Fluke loads of up to 20 000 are usually accompanied by intermittent right upper quadrant pain and tenderness. The most common complication of clonorchiasis is recurrent pyogenic cholangitis, usually secondary to infection with *Escherichia coli*. This is characterized by recurrent attacks of fever and rigors, abdominal pain and jaundice. Both extra- and intrahepatic ducts become dilated and are found to contain soft pigment stones, biliary mud or pus. Intrahepatic bile duct strictures may also develop and contribute to the cholestasis. Worms present in the pancreatic duct can lead to episodes of pancreatitis. Chronic infection is associated with the development of cholangiocarcinoma.

Diagnosis

The diagnosis is most commonly made by finding ova in the stool or worms and ova in biliary drainage. Bile obtained at endoscopic examination or on the sticky string of an Enterotest capsule can be examined for eggs.

Cholangiographic examination can be suggestive of the diagnosis by demonstrating the flukes as uniformly small filling defects and the associated intrahepatic ductal dilatation, strictures and intrahepatic pigment stones.

Immunodiagnostic tests are available but cross-reactions with other trematodes are common.

Treatment

Praziquantel in a dose of 25 mg/kg tds given on two consecutive days gives a high cure rate. For chronic advanced disease surgical exploration and drainage of the common bile duct is sometimes required.

Prevention and control

In areas where the two intermediate hosts are found and raw fish is frequently consumed contamination of fish culture ponds by human and animal faeces must be minimized. Night soil can be stored at 4 to 8 °C for 5 days to kill the eggs. Measures aimed at reducing infection include killing the metacercariae by thorough cooking, by freezing at −10 °C for 5 days, or by storing in a 10% saline solution for longer than one day. Most of these procedures are not practical where the infection is endemic.

Opisthorciasis

Aetiology and epidemiology

Opisthorciasis is caused by two very similar flukes, namely *Opisthorcis felineus* and *O. viverrini*. These parasites are morphologically very similar to *C. sinensis* and produce a similar clinical picture. *O. felineus*, a parasite of cats and other animals, is found in man in East Prussia, Poland and Siberia and occasionally in India. *O. viverrini* is found in up to 25% of the population of north-eastern Thailand. The life cycle is the same as *C. sinensis* with a definitive mammalian host and snail and freshwater fish intermediate hosts.

Clinical features
In endemic areas infection begins early in life and usually remains asymptomatic until around the fifth decade when repeated infections have given rise to a significant worm burden. An acute syndrome of irregular high fever, lymphadenopathy, myalgia, arthralgia, skin eruptions and occasional facial oedema has been described but appears uncommon. In chronic longstanding infections symptoms are much the same as with *C. sinensis*. An association with cholangiocarcinoma has been reported in Thailand.

Diagnosis
The diagnosis is made by finding *Opisthorcis* eggs in faeces or bile. Eggs cannot be easily distinguished from those of *Chlonorchis*. The egg count does not relate to worm burden and often drops with increasing parasite load.

Treatment
Praziquantel is the treatment of choice. A single doze of 50 mg/kg has been demonstrated to give a cure rate of 97% in heavy infections whilst 25 mg/kg tds for one day is reported to be 100% successful.

Prevention and control
Educating people to change the habits of a lifetime and not eat raw or undercooked fish is not often productive. Improving sanitation and preventing contamination of fish ponds with human faeces is helpful. Mass treatment has had some success in control programmes in Thailand.

Fasciola hepatica

Aetiology and epidemiology
Fascioliasis is an infection caused by the sheep liver fluke *Fasciola hepatica*, and has a worldwide distribution, being particularly common in sheep-rearing areas.

Adult *F. hepatica* live in the large biliary ducts of sheep, goats and cattle, and occasionally in man who is an accidental host. The adult fluke measures up to 3 cm in length and 1.2 cm in breadth and is brownish in colour. Large, ovoid eggs (140 × 80 μm) are passed in the host faeces. A miracidium hatches in water within 3 weeks and penetrates a lymnaeid snail where it develops through rediae and daughter rediae stages to cercariae. The cercariae emerge from the snail and encyst on various aquatic vegetation to develop into metacercariae. Infection occurs when a suitable mammalian host ingests infected vegetation. Human infection is often related to consumption of watercress. The metacercariae excyst in the duodenum, penetrate the intestinal wall and enter the peritoneal cavity. They invade the liver, causing considerable damage, as they migrate to the bile ducts.

Clinical features

Human fascioliasis is usually mild. During the migratory phase upper gastrointestinal symptoms of nausea, vomiting and epigastric and right hypochondrial pain, fever and urticaria associated with marked eosinophilia may occur. Once flukes reach the bile ducts there are few symptoms, although rarely a fluke may block the common bile duct. Flukes occasionally migrate to ectopic sites and give rise to pruritic painful nodules or abscesses. In Lebanon and Syria adult worms ingested in raw liver may attach themselves to the pharyngeal mucosa, causing a marked local allergic reaction, in a condition known as halzoun.

Diagnosis

Diagnosis is based on finding the eggs in the stool. The eggs may be difficult to distinguish from those of *Fasciolopsis buski*. Serological investigation is particularly helpful in the migratory phase of the illness, before eggs are produced.

Treatment

Praziquantel is effective when give at a dose of 25 mg/kg three times daily for 2 days.

Prevention and control

Human fascioliasis is prevented by not eating fresh aquatic plants, by boiling drinking water and by thoroughly cooking sheep and goat liver.

INTESTINAL FLUKES IN MAN

Intestinal flukes are zoonoses and man is accidentally infected. More than 50 species have been reported in man and include *Fasciolopsis buski, Heterophyes heterophyes, Metagonimus yokogawai,*

Gastrodiscoides hominis and *Echinostoma*. It is estimated that some 50 million people harbour one or more species of these flukes.

Fasciolopsis buski

Aetiology and epidemiology

Fasciolopsis buski is normally a parasite of pigs which form the reservoir for this infection. Fasciolopsiasis is found in the Far East where the infection is endemic in China and has a more limited distribution in Taiwan, Malaysia, Laos, Burma, Bangladesh and Assam. The adult fluke is found in the small intestine and grows up to 75 mm long and 20 mm wide, being ovoid in shape and up to 3 mm thick. It is flesh coloured and has an oral and ventral sucker. Eggs are produced which are 140 × 80 µm, oval, yellowish brown, with a clear thin outer shell and an operculated end. Eggs are passed out in the faeces from which miracidia develop to enter the first intermediate host, the snail. Cercariae are released from the snail and encyst on water plants. Man ingests the encysted metacercariae on these freshwater plants and they excyst in the duodenum, attach themselves to the intestinal mucosa, and develop into mature adults. Edible water plants involved include water caltrop, water chestnut, water bamboo and watercress.

Clinical features

Most infections are light and asymptomatic. Inflammation and ulceration at the site of attachment gives rise to abdominal pain and diarrhoea. Malabsorption may develop and a protein-losing enteropathy leads to oedema, ascites and cachexia. Heavy fluke burden has been described as leading to intestinal obstruction.

Diagnosis

Diagnosis is usually made on finding the eggs in faeces. The adult flukes are short lived and a diagnosis unlikely in a patient who has been away from an endemic area for over 6 months.

Treatment

The treatment of choice is praziquantel in a single dose of 15 mg/kg given on retiring to bed. The dead flukes will be expelled on the following day.

Prevention and control
Prevention and control involves avoidance of pig manure as fertilizer in areas where edible water plants are cultivated. Cooking and drying of water plants destroys the metacercariae. Snail control with chemical molluscicides and mass treatment programmes have also proven to be effective in control.

Heterophyiasis

Aetiology and epidemiology
Of the ten or more minute heterophyid flukes which have been found in man *Heterophyes heterophyes* is the most common. Human infection is common in Egypt, Iran and areas of the Far East including China, South Korea and the Philippines. The fluke inhabits the small intestine of humans and a variety of fish-eating mammals. Snails are the first intermediate hosts of this fluke and freshwater or brackish water fish the second intermediate hosts. Man acquires the fluke by eating infected raw fish.

Clinical features
Adult flukes can cause inflammation and ulceration of the small intestinal mucosa and heavy infections give rise to symptoms of dyspepsia and mucous diarrhoea. Eggs, similar in size to those of *Clonorchis sinensis*, are deposited in the bowel wall and may enter blood vessels and reach the heart or central nervous system and result in cardiac failure or epilepsy.

Diagnosis
The diagnosis is based on the identification of eggs in the stool. These must be differentiated from those of *Clonorchis* and other heterophyid trematodes. The infection dies out naturally within two years of leaving an endemic area.

Treatment
Praziquantel in a dose of 20 mg/kg daily for 3 days has been demonstrated to produce a 100% cure.

Prevention and control
The basis for prevention and control is the same as that for clonorchiasis.

Metagonimiasis

Aetiology and epidemiology
Metagonimus yokogawai is a small fluke (1–2.5 mm) which inhabits the small intestine of man and fish-eating mammals and some birds. It is endemic in China, Taiwan, Korea and Japan. The life cycle and intermediate hosts are similar to *Heterophyes*.

Clinical features
Clinical manifestations are those found with *Heterophyes*, but ectopic egg deposition is less commonly a problem.

Diagnosis
The diagnosis is based on recovery of eggs from the stool.

Treatment
Praziquantel is the treatment of choice given as a single dose of 20 mg/kg.

Prevention and control
Prevention is as for clonorchiasis and heterophyiasis.

Gastrodisciasis

Aetiology and epidemiology
The fluke *Gastroidiscoides hominis* inhabits the large intestine of man and is commonly found in Assam, Bengal and Bihar in India and has been reported from Malaysia, Indonesia, Thailand and the Philippines. The adult produces greenish brown eggs not dissimilar to those of *F. buski*. The first intermediate host is a snail from which cercariae emerge to encyst as metacercariae on freshwater plants.

Clinical features
Most infections are asymptomatic, although with heavy infections mucous diarrhoea may occur.

Diagnosis
The diagnosis is based on finding the characteristic ova in the faeces.

Treatment
Praziquantel in a single dose of 15 mg/kg appears to be effective.

Prevention and control
Thorough cooking of edible vegetation will prevent infection.

Echinostomiasis

Aetiology and epidemiology
Echinostoma is an intestinal fluke of birds and mammals. Some 12 species have been reported as occasional parasites of man. Infection can arise in areas with a combination of factors including an abundance of freshwater snails, which can act as primary and secondary intermediate hosts, and molluscs, which are sometimes found to be secondary intermediate hosts, poor sanitary conditions, and man's propensity for a diet of uncooked snails and molluscs. The infection is most commonly found in Indonesia, Philippines and Thailand.

Clinical features
Only in heavy infections do these small intestinal flukes give rise to symptoms of diarrhoea and abdominal discomfort.

Diagnosis
Eggs, similar to but smaller than those of *F. buski*, may be found in the stool.

Treatment
Praziquantel in a single dose of 25 mg/kg may be effective.

Prevention and control
Thorough cooking or avoidance of the culinary delights of uncooked snails and molluscs will minimize the risk of infection.

LUNG FLUKES OR PARAGONIMIASIS

Aetiology and epidemiology

Paragonimus westermani is the most common and widespread of the 13 species of fluke known to cause disease in man. Infection in man is not uncommon in areas of the Far East, including China, Japan, Taiwan, Korea and the Philippines. Other species of *Paragonimus* are known to infect man in the Far East, Africa and Central and South America. The definitive hosts of the *Paragonimus* fluke are normally wild carnivores.

The adult fluke is oval, reddish-brown and translucent, measuring some 10–20 × 5–10 mm. Adult flukes live in cystic cavities in the lungs and produce eggs which are discharged into the bronchi and are coughed out in sputum or swallowed to be passed out in the faeces. To continue their development the eggs must reach water inhabited by the first intermediate host, a freshwater snail. Miracidiae emerging from the eggs invade these freshwater snails where they undergo development into cercariae. These cercariae emerge to invade the second intermediate host, a suitable freshwater crab or crayfish. Metacercariae develop within the flesh of this intermediate host. When the raw infected crustacean is eaten by the definitive host the metacercariae excyst in the jejunum, penetrate the intestinal wall and enter the peritoneal cavity. Further development takes place within various abdominal organs, including the bowel wall and the liver, before the parasite penetrates the diaphragm to reach the pleural cavity and lung. Adult flukes have been known to live for 10 to 20 years.

Man acquires the fluke by eating raw infected crabs or crayfish or foods prepared with or cross-contaminated by their flesh or juices. In some mammalian hosts the larval fluke cannot mature and remains at a larval stage in the muscles. Eating the raw flesh of wild boar infected in this manner has led to disease in man.

Clinical features

The adult flukes usually settle in the lung close to the pleura causing local lung necrosis, an inflammatory exudate and eventual fibrous encapsulation. Eggs trapped within the lung elicit a granulomatous reaction resembling that of a tubercle. Flukes may migrate from the lung to almost any tissue.

Pulmonary paragonimiasis

Most light and moderate infections are asymptomatic. Symptoms may become apparent up to 2 years after infection. Commonly there is a gradual onset of productive cough and chest discomfort. The cough is spasmodic and often related to exercise. The sputum is tenacious and rusty brown due to discoloration by both eggs and blood staining. Frank haemoptysis may occur and can often be the presenting symptom. Episodic pleuritic pain is often a feature and may be associated with pleural effusions. Bronchiectasis and pulmonary fibrosis may develop in chronic infections and be associated with finger clubbing. Secondary bronchopneumonia and lung abscess may develop.

Radiographic changes are often similar to those in tuberculosis with ill-defined shadowing. Unlike tuberculosis apical lesions are uncommon, and lesions due to paragonimiasis are more common in the right lung.

The patient's health is rarely seriously impaired and fatalities are few.

Cerebral and spinal paragonimiasis

The brain is the most common site for invasion when the aberrant migration of flukes occurs. Symptoms are those of a space-occupying lesion. Plain skull X-rays may demonstrate signs of cerebral shift, raised intracranial pressure, or cerebral calcification. The parasitic cysts can be demonstrated by computerized axial tomography. Spinal involvement with both motor and sensory signs is seen occasionally.

Cerebral paragonimiasis carries a 5% mortality. Chronic sequelae include epilepsy, dementia, decreased visual acuity and hemiplegia.

Other ectopic sites

Subcutaneous lesions caused by migrating immature flukes may occur. Firm, tender, slightly mobile nodules, a few centimetres in diameter may be found slowly migrating beneath the skin.

Worm cysts may develop in the intestinal wall giving rise to diarrhoea, which may be bloody. Peritoneal cysts may cause considerable pain and elicit an inflammatory response leading to the formation of adhesions.

Eggs may enter the circulation and be widely disseminated, often lodging in the heart, liver, kidneys and brain, where egg granulomata develop.

Diagnosis

The clinical differential diagnosis of lung paragonimiasis includes tuberculosis, lung abscess and other mass and cystic lesions. Cerebral and spinal paragonimiasis must be distinguished from abscess, tuberculous granulomata and other helminthic infections of the CNS, e.g. schistosomiasis, cysticercosis and hydatid.

The *Paragonimus* egg is brown and asymmetrically ovoid, measuring some $100 \times 60\ \mu m$, having a thick shell and flattened operculum. The diagnosis can be confirmed by finding these characteristic ova in sputum, stool, pleural fluid and CSF, or by finding adult flukes in subcutaneous nodules. Both adults and egg granulomata may be demonstrated in surgical specimens.

Serological tests are often sensitive but lack specificity. These tests will however revert to being negative within 6 months of successful treatment and are useful as a test of cure.

Treatment

The drug of choice is praziquantel at a dose of 25 mg/kg three times daily after food for 3 days. Treatment of cerebral lesions should be under cover of dexamethasone to reduce any cerebral oedema provoked by the dying parasite (cf. cerebral cysticercosis). The cure rate is very high. Depending on the severity and chronicity of the disease a second course of treatment may be required.

Prevention and control

Health education stressing the need to cook all crustacean food and the requirement for the sanitary disposal of sputum and faeces is required in endemic areas. The control of freshwater snails with molluscicides can be performed where feasible.

Part Three
Bacterial Diseases

13
Tuberculosis

INTRODUCTION

The burden of tuberculous disease in the developing world is enormous. The annual incidence of new cases of all forms of tuberculosis is between 7 and 10 million cases. Estimates suggest 2.6 million deaths from tuberculosis every year. Many children die from tuberculous meningitis and miliary tuberculosis, but the greatest burden falls on the adult population: the parents, workers and leaders in society.

EPIDEMIOLOGY AND PATHOGENESIS

Tuberculosis is in the main caused by *Mycobacterium tuberculosis*. The source of tuberculous infection is the patient with pulmonary tuberculosis in whose sputum mycobacteria can be demonstrated. The bacilli are transmitted to close contacts of the patient by droplets discharged when the patient coughs. Inhalation of these droplets by an as yet healthy, uninfected individual will lead to a primary infection, which may be latent. When the bacilli become deposited in the pulmonary alveoli they multiply and form an inflammatory primary focus. From this lesion bacilli may spread by the blood and lymphatics to the rest of the body, especially to the lymph nodes, bones and kidneys. The main lymph nodes to become involved are those which drain the primary lung focus and the two together form what is called the primary complex. In the majority of cases the lesion resolves as the individual mounts an acquired immune response. Widespread disease may however result especially in the young, giving rise to conditions such as miliary tuberculosis or tuberculous meningitis. Occasionally, as hypersensitivity develops, the primary focus may become destructive and extend locally. However in the majority of cases this primary infection is asymptomatic or at worst symptoms are of a trivial nature.

The hypersensitivity which develops during this primary infection greatly alters the response to either endogenous reactivation or exogenous reinfection. Reactivation of the pulmonary focus leads to the formation of granulomata with caseation, often with extensive tissue destruction and necrosis. Cavities may form in the lung, and once these cavities drain into the bronchial system a new source of infection is created. The most commonly affected sites of post-primary tuberculosis are the apical and subapical regions of the lungs, probably because these areas have the highest intra-alveolar oxygen tension, but any of the sites of the original primary haematogenous spread may be involved.

Tubercle bacilli disseminated from or surviving in the primary focus may remain dormant for many years, their multiplication being suppressed by the enhanced immune response. Any condition which compromises this cellular immunity makes reactivation more likely.

PULMONARY TUBERCULOSIS

Primary pulmonary tuberculosis

Clinical features
Primary pulmonary tuberculosis is most often asymptomatic and only presents as a result of routine screening of contacts of an infectious case. Symptoms when present are those of a dry cough, low grade fever and malaise with loss of appetite. Rarely erythema nodosum or phlyctenular keratoconjunctivitis may be seen.

The lymphadenopathy component of the primary complex may be prominent, particularly in young children. Bronchial or tracheal compression may occur and can give rise to paroxysmal coughing or wheeze or can result in lobar or segmental collapse. Erosion of these structures and rupture of nodes into the air passages can lead to severe respiratory embarrassment. Obstructive emphysema or bronchiectasis can develop distal to bronchial obstruction.

Involvement of the pleura in the tuberculous process may elicit a pleural reaction and the development of a pleural effusion.

Diagnosis
The tuberculin test is usually strongly positive. In young children the lymphadenopathy is usually prominent on chest radiographs, whilst in older children and adults the lung component of the primary complex is most obvious, being commonly found in the lower or mid zones close to the pleura. Bacteriological confirmation should be sought by culture of sputum, upper respiratory tract swabs or gastric washings.

Treatment
Therapy should be given to prevent local complications and further dissemination. Unless the possibility of resistant organisms is a concern, then a two drug regimen is sufficient. One suggested regimen is rifampicin 10 mg/kg daily in combination with isoniazid 5–10 mg/kg daily. Treatment is given for 9 months. If a third drug is required because of the possibility of drug resistance then streptomycin 20 mg/kg per day may be given parenterally for the first two months of the treatment regimen. Ethambutol, with its potential for eye toxicity, should not be given to children too young to report visual symptoms.

Post-primary pulmonary tuberculosis

Clinical features
The course of post-primary pulmonary tuberculosis varies between a chronic, low grade disease with a balance between lung cavitation and healing by fibrosis, through to fulminant disease with rapid and gross pulmonary cavitation.

Early symptoms of pulmonary tuberculosis include general malaise, weight loss, fever and night sweats. Respiratory symptoms include cough, which when productive appears purulent and sometimes bloodstained. Chest pain, often a non-specific discomfort and sometimes pleuritic in nature, is a common complaint.

Release of material from a tuberculous lesion into the pleural space will provoke a marked inflammatory reaction and the formation of a pleural effusion. Rupture of a cavity or large caseating lesion into the pleural space will give rise to the development of an empyema or pyopneumothorax associated with a bronchopleural fistula.

Blood staining of the sputum arises from ulceration of the bronchial mucosa. When a pulmonary arterial vessel is eroded by a tuberculous cavity there may be profound and sometimes fatal haemoptysis.

Tuberculous laryngitis may occur in patients who are coughing up bacilli and presents with hoarseness and throat discomfort and occasionally as dysphagia.

Diagnosis

Microscopic examination of the sputum for tubercle bacilli is the quickest way of making a diagnosis. The bacilli are acid-fast and can be seen under the light microscope after Ziehl-Neelsen staining. A more rapid and sensitive technique requiring fluorescence microscopy utilizes staining with auramine O or auramine-rhodamine but may not be readily available in the developing world.

Mycobacteria can be cultured on Lowenstein-Jensen medium. Sputum, laryngeal swabs, gastric aspirates, pleural fluid or pleural biopsies can all be utilized in attempts to culture the bacilli. Once cultured *in vitro* sensitivities to anti-tuberculous drugs can be determined and used when designing a treatment regimen.

The diagnosis of the tuberculous nature of a pleural effusion is best made by obtaining a pleural biopsy by needle aspiration. Histological examination can demonstrate the presence of caseating granulomata, with or without the presence of acid-fast bacilli, and tissue may be submitted for culture for tubercle bacilli. The pleural exudate is usually lymphocytic but rarely contains tubercle bacilli on smear or culture. Direct smear of pus from a tuberculous empyema, however, may well demonstrate the presence of bacilli.

There are no pathognomonic radiographic appearances of pulmonary tuberculosis. The diagnosis is supported by the finding of upper lobe shadowing, particularly in the posterior and apical segments, which may be bilateral or associated with cavitation. Pleural effusions, mediastinal lymphadenopathy, pulmonary nodules or diffuse miliary shadowing may all be radiological features.

Treatment

For the treatment of pulmonary tuberculosis in Britain the British Thoracic Society (BTS) recommends 6 months of treatment with four drugs:

Months 1 and 2: Rifampicin + isoniazid + pyrazinamide + either ethambutol or streptomycin.
Months 3 to 6: Rifampicin and isoniazid.

The fourth drug (streptomycin or ethambutol) probably contributes little and many specialists now successfully give only three drugs.

An alternative regimen also recommended by the BTS is a 9 month regimen:

Months 1 and 2: Rifampicin + isoniazid + either ethambutol or streptomycin.
Months 3 to 9: Rifampicin + isoniazid.

Whilst this is the counsel of perfection it is rarely possible to achieve this in developing countries where resources cannot be found to finance expensive drug regimens and the compliance of unsupervised patients may well be less than perfect.

The least expensive regimen is a combination of isoniazid with thiacetazone given daily for at least one year with the addition of streptomycin for the first 2 months of treatment. The usual dose regimen is isoniazid 300 mg, thiacetazone 150 mg and streptomycin 0.75 mg to 1 g daily. By virtue of the need to administer the streptomycin parenterally the first two months of this treatment are supervised. The length of the course of treatment and the common and unpleasant side-effects of thiacetazone lead however to poor compliance and increased drop-out rate. Where regular access to a medical facility with close monitoring of compliance is not logistically possible then direct supervision of the patient's drug intake should ideally be performed by someone, be it a village 'health care worker' or village elder.

Currently efforts are being directed to identifying shorter, effective treatment regimens, ideally including rifampicin/pyrazinamide, which are less expensive and conducive to better compliance. After an initial period of intensive treatment these regimens can incorporate a maintenance phase whereby treatment may be given intermittently on a supervised twice weekly basis, again reducing cost and improving compliance.

Prevention and control
It is now generally accepted that the combination of case-finding and antituberculous chemotherapy is the most important compo-

nent of a tuberculosis control programme and that the roles of chemoprophylaxis and BCG vaccination are subsidiary. The most important group of people in this context are those with pulmonary tuberculosis and who have cough with sputum which is smear-positive, because these are the infectious cases who spread disease. Active case finding in the community has been attempted by a number of groups. A case definition is often difficult to supply when case finding takes place in communities with a high prevalence of cough. Cases found by actively searching in the community will often admit to having attended a health care facility with respiratory symptoms in the recent past and remain undiagnosed. Facilities are required to ensure that when patients attend at any health facility with complaints of cough or sputum a diagnosis of smear-positive tuberculosis can be made and a course of antituberculous treatment arranged. The mainstay of such a programme is a reliable microscopy service, backed up where possible by facilities for mycobacterial culture. Radiological facilities are expensive, depend upon a supply of electricity and technological know-how, and require proper interpretation of the radiograph if patients are not to be given unnecessary antituberculous treatment.

In order to protect children from developing tuberculosis it is desirable for them to receive BCG vaccination as early in life as possible. In developing countries BCG vaccination forms part of the WHO Expanded Programme of Vaccination and aims for the widest possible coverage. The programme is fraught with organizational and administrative difficulties and cover in many endemic areas is still far from satisfactory.

LYMPH NODE TUBERCULOSIS

Epidemiology and pathogenesis

Lymph node tuberculosis, occurring predominantly in the cervical region, is the most common manifestation of non-respiratory tuberculosis worldwide.

Mycobacterium tuberculosis is the most frequent causative organism. Atypical mycobacteria such as M. *scrofulaceum* and M. *avium-intracellulare* are occasionally found, particularly in cervical lymph node tuberculosis in young children.

Lymph node tuberculosis may occur as a result of primary infection or by extension from a contiguous focus, but is thought by most to be part of a generalized lymphatic and haematogenous spread of tuberculous disease rather than a purely localized disease process. The vast majority of the primary lesions heal and lymphatic tuberculosis is due to a reactivation of a focus of disease. Supraclavicular lymph node tuberculosis is usually secondary to lymphatic spread from mediastinal disease.

Clinical features

In populations where tuberculosis is endemic, tuberculous lymphadenitis has its greatest incidence in early childhood, but occurs in later adulthood in populations where the incidence of tuberculosis is lower.

Cervical node involvement (scrofula) is commonest and accounts for 70% of all lymph node tuberculosis. It is associated with other demonstrable foci of tuberculosis, in the lungs or elsewhere, in about half the cases. The lymph node swelling is usually of insidious onset and is painless, although it may be tender early in the infection when it is enlarging most rapidly. Initially, the lymph nodes are discrete and firm but later they become matted together and fluctuant. The overlying skin may break down with formation of abscesses and chronic discharging sinuses which may heal with scarring.

Between one third to two thirds of patients have constitutional symptoms with fever, night sweats, weight loss and malaise.

Tuberculous lymphadenitis in an immunosuppressed patient may be acute and resemble an acute pyogenic bacterial infection.

Hilar and paratracheal lymph node enlargement is seen in post-primary tuberculosis in some Asian and African ethnic groups. Mediastinal abscesses may occur with involvement of trachea, bronchi and superior vena cava and require urgent surgical intervention. Oesophageal symptoms are uncommon although painful dysphagia has been reported.

Diagnosis

The age, ethnic group and typical clinical features of a patient may suggest the diagnosis of lymph node tuberculosis, as may a positive chest radiograph (in about 50%) and a positive tuberculin skin reaction (present in 90% or more). A definite diagnosis however requires demonstration of *M. tuberculosis* in the pus from draining sinuses or smear, culture and histology of lymph nodes.

Acid-fast bacilli can be demonstrated in one quarter to one half of lymph node biopsy smears. The isolation rate on culture from biopsy or aspirated pus is about 60 to 70%. This relatively low isolation rate probably reflects a very small population of organisms within the lymph nodes, which become enlarged as a result of a hypersensitivity response to tuberculoprotein. Histologically, tuberculous lymphadenitis may show mild reactive hyperplasia or granulomata, usually with caseation and necrosis.

For mediastinal lymph node tuberculosis, which is commonly associated with pulmonary disease, sputum may show acid-fast bacilli even if pulmonary infiltrates are not apparent. The diagnosis can be confirmed by lymph node smear, culture and histology of biopsies obtained by mediastinoscopy, although in areas endemic for tuberculosis, radiographic and clinical features and a strongly positive tuberculin test make the diagnosis so likely that biopsy confirmation is usually not needed.

The main clinical differential diagnoses include lymphoma, carcinomatous metastases and sarcoidosis.

Treatment

A 9 month regimen of isoniazid plus rifampicin supplemented by ethambutol, streptomycin or pyrazinamide in the first 8 weeks is recommended as effective therapy for superficial lymph node tuberculosis.

Lymph nodes may increase in size and new nodes may appear both during and after chemotherapy without indicating a failure of treatment or relapse. These nodes are sterile on culture and their enlargement or reappearance may be due to hypersensitivity to tuberculoprotein released from disrupted macrophages and does not indicate an unfavourable outcome.

TUBERCULOSIS OF THE PERICARDIUM

Epidemiology and pathogenesis

Tuberculosis of the pericardium is rare in developed countries but continues to be important in immunosuppressed patients and in some Asian and African populations. For example, in Transkei and the surrounding regions of south-east Africa, it is one of the commonest causes of congestive heart failure.

Pericarditis usually develops as a result of rupture of a mediastinal lymph node into the pericardial cavity, although lymphhaematogenous spread, and contiguous spread from a primary tuberculous pneumonia, particularly in children, may also occur. Acute pericarditis appears to be a primary allergic response, whereas chronic pericardial effusion and pericardial constriction both reflect granulomatous lesions often with fibrosis and calcification in the later stage.

Clinical features

Tuberculous pericarditis usually presents insidiously with fever, night sweats, malaise, substernal dull pain, tachycardia and pericardial friction rub. The course is, however, acute and fulminant in up to 25% of cases. When pericardial effusion develops, and particularly when tamponade is present, there is dyspnoea, low pulse pressure with pulsus paradoxus, raised jugular venous pressure, hypotension, hepatomegaly and peripheral oedema.

Chronic constrictive pericarditis may occur weeks or years after the acute stage despite treatment. In many Asian and African populations it commonly occurs early in the disease and may be the presenting feature with dyspnoea, weight loss, very high venous pressure, small quiet heart, paradoxical pulse, hepatomegaly, ascites and peripheral oedema.

Diagnosis

Tuberculous pericarditis should be suspected in patients with insidious fever and signs of pericardial effusion, particularly those who are susceptible to tuberculosis.

ECG changes are non-specific but widespread T-wave changes and low-voltage QRS complexes occur and the chest radiograph shows an enlarged cardiac silhouette, with pleural effusions in about half the patients. Chest radiographs may show active pulmonary tuberculosis in 30% of cases. In chronic constrictive pericarditis the heart size is not enlarged and calcification may be seen in the pericardium, particularly on a lateral film.

On echocardiography, pericardial effusion, frank or loculated, or amorphous pericardial material may be demonstrated, depending on the predominant lesion. The heart is relatively immobile. The pericardial fluid commonly contains mostly lymphocytes, but neutrophils may predominate early in acute cases.

Raised adenosine deaminase activity in pericardial fluid may be of value in the early diagnosis of tuberculous pericarditis.

The definitive diagnosis of tuberculous pericarditis can be made by pericardial fluid culture (in up to 59% of cases) or by pericardial histology, where tuberculous granulomata are seen in 70% of pericardial biopsy specimens.

Treatment

With the advent of effective chemotherapy, mortality from tuberculous pericarditis has fallen to less than 30%. A recent controlled study in Transkei has shown that a 6 month regimen consisting of isoniazid plus rifampicin, supplemented by streptomycin and pyrazinamide in the initial 14 weeks, was effective in tuberculous pericarditis. Complete open drainage on admission abolished the need for pericardiocentesis but did not influence the need for pericardiectomy for subsequent constriction or the risk of death. This study also showed that in patients with constriction, prednisolone given in tapering dose (starting 30–60 mg daily, depending on age) for 11 weeks in addition to antituberculous chemotherapy increased the rate of improvement, and probably decreased the risk of death and the need for pericardiectomy. In patients with effusion, prednisolone reduced the risk of death and the need for repeat pericardiocentesis or open surgical drainage. Whether steroid therapy will reduce late constriction or death in the long term is being assessed in a continuing follow-up in Transkei.

ABDOMINAL TUBERCULOSIS

Epidemiology

In many developing nations, abdominal tuberculosis is still commonly seen. With the widespread pasteurization of milk in technically advanced countries, *M. bovis* is no longer a significant cause of abdominal tuberculosis. The most frequently isolated mycobacterium is *M. tuberculosis*. However, *M. avium-intracellulare* can be the causative organism in patients with AIDS, often as part of a disseminated infection.

Clinical features

Tuberculosis can infect any part of the gut from the mouth to the anus. Upper gastrointestinal involvement is relatively rare. Most tuberculous lesions of the upper gastrointestinal tract present either as gastrointestinal bleeding or with pain. Tuberculous lesions in the oesophagus may present with dysphagia and on endoscopy the lesion may resemble an ulcerating tumour. The diagnosis is usually made on histology of specimens obtained endoscopically or at laparotomy and is often an unexpected finding.

Ileo-caecal tuberculosis is a relatively common form of tuberculous enteritis and accounts for between 68 and 85% of all tuberculous lesions of the gut. The terminal ileum is thickened and the whole circumference of the bowel is usually involved, giving rise to a mass in the right iliac fossa. On macroscopic examination the bowel may be indistinguishable from Crohn's disease and strictures may mimic those observed in lymphoma and ischaemia. Adjacent lymph nodes may be enlarged and be either firm or fleshy in character, occasionally with abscess formation, or even calcification. The colon is occasionally involved and may present with gastrointestinal bleeding.

The symptoms of abdominal tuberculosis are often non-specific and insidious in onset, although occasionally the presentation is one of acute abdominal pain. Obstruction, perforation or fistula formation may occur and are associated with a relatively poorer prognosis. Rarely, the presentation may be one of acute appendicitis.

Disseminated infection of the peritoneal cavity (tuberculous peritonitis) may result from ingestion of mycobacteria, local extension of tuberculous disease from the gut into lymphatics, or from haematogenous spread. Tuberculous salpingitis may spread to generalized peritonitis.

In the peritoneal cavity there is frequently ascites and white tubercles scattered throughout the omentum, bowel wall and other organs. The mesentery is often thickened and oedematous and there may be collections of pus or caseous masses. Signs of perforation, obstruction or fistula formation may be apparent. Tuberculous peritonitis usually presents with ascites as a prominent feature with the accompanying symptoms of fever, abdominal distension and weight loss, with or without chronic abdominal pain.

Diagnosis

A high index of suspicion is required to facilitate the diagnosis of abdominal tuberculosis in view of the great diversity of clinical presentations it affords.

Fever is common and approximately 50% of patients have abdominal distension or ascites. Abdominal tenderness and hepatomegaly are less common. In the case of ileo-caecal tuberculosis there may be a palpable mass in the right iliac fossa and indeed abdominal masses may be palpated in any part of the abdomen due to loops of bowel that are matted together, and may give rise to the classical description of a 'doughy' abdomen.

Routine haematological investigations may reveal non-specific findings such as raised erythrocyte sedimentation rate (ESR) and anaemia. Most patients have a normal white cell count. The tuberculin test is often not helpful and falsely negative, particularly in the elderly, the undernourished and those with disseminated disease.

Ascitic fluid in tuberculous peritonitis is usually an exudate with a protein content in excess of 3.5 g/dl, most often clear and straw-coloured and commonly with more than 300 white cells/ml with a lymphocyte predominance. Ziehl-Neelsen staining and culture for *M. tuberculosis* is often negative.

Chest radiographs will demonstrate evidence of tuberculous infection in about 50% of patients. Plain abdominal radiographs may reveal the presence of ascites and there may be distended small bowel loops with fluid levels seen on the erect film. Barium examination may reveal features of ileo-caecal involvement. Lesions of the colon may be single or multiple and have an annular appearance with shouldering, similar to the features of colonic carcinoma. Colonoscopy combined with biopsy and examination of colonoscopic brushings can aid diagnosis in this situation.

Ultrasound and computerized tomographic (CT) scanning have emerged as helpful non-invasive methods of investigation. Both methods may show features that are highly suggestive (but not pathognomonic) of tuberculous peritonitis and/or gastrointestinal involvement. Scans will demonstrate ascites, lymphadenopathy, thickened mesentery and irregular soft tissue densities in the omentum and central caseation can sometimes be demonstrated in lymph nodes with CT scanning.

Definitive diagnosis of tuberculous peritonitis requires either culture of the organism or a biopsy specimen of peritoneum, gut or lymph node showing the characteristic histological appearances of caseating granulomas or acid-fast bacilli. Laparotomy will confirm the diagnosis in nearly every patient but is a major invasive procedure. Blind percutaneous needle biopsy of peritoneum has been employed with variable success in obtaining diagnostic material. Open peritoneal biopsy is probably safer and more reliable and avoids the potential risk of perforating bowel. However, laparoscopy with peritoneal biopsy has been described as effective and safe, and hence is the investigation of choice where available.

Other methods for obtaining rapid diagnosis of abdominal tuberculosis have been reported and include measurement of ascitic fluid adenosine deaminase activity and an enzyme-linked immunosorbent assay (ELISA) to detect circulating IgG antibodies to *M. tuberculosis*.

Treatment

Controlled clinical trials of drug regimens for tuberculous peritonitis have not been conducted and very few reports of long-term follow-up have been reported. With modern treatment the prognosis is generally favourable, providing the patient does not suffer potentially lethal complications such as gastrointestinal bleeding, perforation or infarction. Even with these complications, the prognosis may be favourable with skilled surgical management. Ideally patients should receive four antituberculous drugs initially, namely isoniazid, rifampicin, pyrazinamide and either streptomycin or ethambutol, in dosages that are employed for pulmonary tuberculosis. Isoniazid and rifampicin are given for a total of 9 months and the companion drugs are usually given for 2 or 4 months depending on progress.

The use of cortiscosteroid drugs in the treatment of tuberculous peritonitis is controversial. There is the theoretical value of reducing inflammation and fibrosis and promoting prompt resolution of ascitic fluid. However, unlike tuberculous pericarditis and pleural effusion for which corticosteroids have been shown to speed up resolution and improve prognosis, there are few such reports for tuberculous peritonitis.

GENITOURINARY TUBERCULOSIS

Renal tuberculosis does not usually manifest itself until adult life. Early lesions occur in the renal cortex. Tuberculous cavities in the renal parenchyma can rupture into the renal pelvis and result in spread of infection down the ureter to the bladder. Ureteric obstruction may result and give rise to hydronephrosis. Tuberculosis of the bladder results in ulceration, fibrosis and shrinkage. Genital tuberculosis in the male is usually secondary to renal tract infection, but the association is less common in the female.

Clinical features

Renal tuberculosis may present with frank or microscopic haematuria, loin and back pain, and ureteric colic. In advanced disease there may be evidence of impairment of renal function, often secondary to hydronephrosis, rather than tuberculous destruction of the kidney per se. A cold abscess may develop in the loin in advanced disease. The commonest presenting features of tuberculous cystitis are frequency and dysuria. Tuberculosis of the male genital tract may involve the epididymis, testis, seminal vesicles or prostate. The usual clinical finding is a scrotal mass that may be tender or associated with a draining sinus. In the female the fallopian tubes and endometrium are the usual sites of infection. Symptoms are usually local consisting of menstrual disorders, sub-fertility and abdominal pain. The presenting symptoms may be those of pelvic inflammatory disease unresponsive to antibiotic therapy.

Treatment

Antituberculous chemotherapy is given on the lines of that used for pulmonary tuberculosis. In the presence of renal impairment both streptomycin and ethambutol should be used with caution. Corticosteroids have a role in the management of ureteric obstruction and are often helpful in reducing the distressing symptoms of cystitis.

TUBERCULOSIS OF THE SPINE

Epidemiology

Tuberculosis of the spine is the commonest manifestation of orthopaedic tuberculosis. The condition is a rare form of extrapulmonary tuberculosis, but, in many developing nations, is a significant cause of crippling deformities.

Clinical features

The most common presentation of tuberculosis of the spine is of back pain of variable duration. Most patients have had symptoms for some months, occasionally even years. Rarely there may be radicular pain which may be referred to the loin or abdomen and may be mistaken for an abdominal condition. There may be lower limb symptoms or sphincter disturbance due to cord compression by associated abscess formation.

Examination may reveal local tenderness or muscular spasm and mild kyphosis. In more advanced cases there may be gross kyphosis at presentation. If there is associated psoas abscess formation, a fluctuant mass may appear in the groin. Large psoas abscesses may occasionally be palpated abdominally.

Diagnosis

Tuberculous infections of the spine often start as a discitis of the intervertebral disc and then spread along the anterior and longitudinal ligaments to involve the adjacent vertebral bodies. Hence on plain X-ray films of the spine the anterior edges of superior and inferior borders of adjacent vertebral bodies are often eroded with narrowing of the disc space. There is progressive destruction of the vertebral bodies with loss of height and subsequent kyphosis. Occasionally more than one disc space may be involved and lesions may 'skip' with healthy vertebrae in between. The lower thoracic, lumbar and lumbo-sacral vertebrae are the sites most commonly involved. Infections of the cervical vertebrae are relatively rare. Paravertebral abscess formation is a common complication of spinal tuberculosis.

In a patient with evidence of pulmonary tuberculosis and a suggestive spinal lesion, it is often unnecessary to confirm the diagnosis by invasive investigations of the spinal site. The differential diagnosis includes malignancy and other pyogenic spinal infections. Malignant spinal metastases tend to erode the pedicles and spinal bodies and leave the disc intact, in contrast to tuberculous infections which erode the disc early in the disease process. The onset of pyogenic infections is often more acute and the pain may be more severe. Invasive procedures either by needle biopsy or by open exploration may be undertaken to establish a firm diagnosis and it is important that all specimens are collected not only for histology, but also for culture for both pyogenic organisms and for *M. tuberculosis*.

Treatment

Ambulatory short-course chemotherapy has been proven to be highly effective in the treatment of tuberculosis of the spine and for the great majority of the patients operative procedures are unnecessary. Short course regimens of isoniazid plus rifampicin for 6 to 9 months are highly effective in the treatment of tuberculosis of the spine. No additional benefit derives from bed rest, a plaster jacket or debridement operations. Patients who develop acute cord compression may require early surgical intervention.

TUBERCULOUS MENINGITIS

Aetiology and epidemiology

Tuberculous meningitis (TBM) is an important problem in areas endemic for tuberculosis, particularly because late diagnosis or inadequate treatment may result in permanent disability, neurological sequelae, or death. The incidence of meningeal involvement reflects the overall prevalence of tuberculosis in the community. In India, TBM is the commonest form of meningitis.

Tuberculous meningitis usually arises as a complication, immediate or remote, of the primary infection. Bacilli gain access to the cerebro-spinal fluid (CSF) after rupture of small caseous microtubercles in the meninges or subpial tuberculomas in the brain or spinal column.

Clinical features

Involvement of the meninges and nervous system by tuberculosis is usually preceded by 2–8 weeks' history of non-specific symptoms of malaise, fatigue, anorexia, headache, nausea and vomiting. Children may become irritable, drowsy or develop behavioural disorders. There is usually a low grade fever which rarely exceeds 39 °C. Neck stiffness in TBM is rarely marked.

Papilloedema is common and may be present without headache, hydrocephalus, raised intracranial pressure or impaired visual acuity. The presence of choroid tubercles can help in diagnosis. Visual failure may develop due to opto-chiasmatic arachnoiditis or tuberculoma compressing the optic nerve or chiasma. Cranial nerve palsies are found in up to one third of patients. Oculomotor nerve palsies (III and VI) are common and the only evidence may be large pupils which react slowly to light. Rarely, internuclear ophthalmoplegia and horizontal gaze pareses develop, and indicate intrinsic brain stem dysfunction and a poor prognosis. Other cranial nerves which are commonly involved are the VIIth and VIIIth nerves.

As the disease progresses, focal neurological signs may appear, including mono- or hemiparesis, cerebellar signs, extrapyramidal and hypothalamic disturbances. Raised intracranial pressure may develop as a result of either cerebral oedema, obstructive hydrocephalus or expanding intracranial tuberculomas.

Epileptic seizures may occur, particularly in children. Seizures developing months after the start of chemotherapy may indicate the development of a cerebral tuberculoma. Hyponatraemia due to inappropriate antidiuretic hormone secretion may also be a cause of central nervous system dysfunction.

The brunt of TBM may fall on the spinal meninges resulting in 'spinal TB meningitis' with signs of a myeloradiculopathy. Patients have severe flaccid or spastic tetraplegia, with early loss of sphincter function. There may be little or no cerebral symptoms or signs. The CSF protein is nearly always raised with values up to 100 times normal. Return of useful function is infrequent. Potts disease or paraspinal abscess are usually accompanied by more pain but must be excluded.

Diagnosis

Routine blood tests are not particularly helpful in diagnosis. The white cell count and erythrocyte sedimentation rate are often normal. Hyponatraemia due to inappropriate ADH secretion may be present. The tuberculin skin test may be absent or depressed in disseminated tuberculosis. Chest radiographic evidence of active tuberculosis is of great diagnostic importance.

Lumbar puncture will demonstrate a raised CSF opening pressure. The CSF cell count is increased but is usually under $500/mm^3$. Characteristically, lymphocytes predominate, although in 15% of patients, polymorphonuclear leukocytes may predominate early in the infection. The CSF protein is usually elevated. CSF glucose concentrations are generally low but may occasionally be normal.

146 Tuberculosis

The direct smear examination of CSF for acid-fast bacilli is often negative. A positive culture is obtained in only about half of the patients. The first CSF specimen is the most likely one to be culture positive. The yield of positive cultures from CSF may be improved by the use of selective Kirchner culture medium. The bromide partition test, CSF complement, C reactive protein, immunoglobulin and adenosine deaminase levels all hold no advantages over conventional CSF criteria in the diagnosis of TBM and do not differentiate bacterial from tuberculous infections. Estimation of antibody titres to the tubercle bacillus, purified protein derivative, and to antigen 5 to *M. tuberculosis* have been employed in an attempt to improve the early diagnosis of TBM. A more sensitive and specific recently described test is detection of tuberculostearic acid, a structural component of *M. tuberculosis* by gas chromatography with mass spectroscopy. Other antigens can be detected using ELISA or latex particle agglutination technique. When these tests become commercially available, the rapid diagnosis of TBM will be greatly facilitated as they are rapid and reliable and require only small volumes of CSF.

CT scanning is very helpful in the diagnosis of TBM and demonstrates the characteristic features of contrast enhancement in the basal meninges, as well as cerebral oedema, infarction and intracerebral tuberculomas.

Important differential diagnoses of TBM include partially treated pyogenic meningitis, aseptic lymphocytic meningitis, cryptococcal meningitis, malignant meningitis and cerebral lupus.

Treatment

Treatment is based on quadruple therapy of daily intramuscular streptomycin, oral isoniazid (10 mg/kg), rifampicin (15 mg/kg) and pyrazinamide (35 mg/kg). These drugs form the most bactericidal combination with pyrazinamide and isoniazid, which readily cross the blood–brain barrier, making the largest contribution. Streptomycin crosses the meninges when they are inflamed, but not once the integrity of the blood–brain barrier is restored, and is used for the first two months of the treatment regimen. The remaining three drugs are given for at least one year. Where rifampicin is found to be too expensive, treatment with the remaining three drugs should suffice. Failure to improve or subsequent deterioration early in the course of treatment is most commonly due to the development of hydrocephalus, and requires early surgical intervention. Deterioration later in the course of chemotherapy may be due to an enlarging intracranial tuberculoma. This paradoxical development of intracranial tuberculomas during chemotherapy is due to a hypersensitivity response to tuberculoprotein.

Corticosteroids have been demonstrated to increase survival and reduce long-term sequelae and should be given to all patients with TBM.

TUBERCULOSIS AND HUMAN IMMUNODEFICIENCY VIRUS

The AIDS epidemic has had a profound impact on tuberculosis morbidity and is a particular problem among those demographic groups with a high existing incidence of tuberculosis. The World Health Organization estimated that three million persons had 'dual infection' in 1990 (78% occurring in Africa), and that 3.9% of all cases of tuberculosis worldwide were HIV associated, but that in sub-Saharan Africa this figure was 17%.

Infection with HIV leads to reactivation of latent tuberculous infection. Clinical tuberculosis may be expected to develop in about 30% of HIV positive subjects with past tuberculous infection, and cases will also occur among those who are HIV positive and tuberculin negative and have become susceptible to primary infection. In addition, further cases of tuberculosis may occur through spread to the general non-HIV infected population.

HIV associated pulmonary tuberculosis is significantly more likely to be associated with prolonged diarrhoea, generalized lymphadenopathy and skin rashes before treatment. Pulmonary tuberculosis may be more difficult to establish in HIV infected patients; the chest radiograph is often atypical and sputum smears for acid-fast bacilli may be less sensitive in diagnosis, probably as a result of diminished pulmonary cavitation in this group. Histological examination of tuberculous lesions in patients who are HIV positive demonstrates poorly formed granulomata and little evidence of caseous necrosis. This anergic non-reactive histology is also reflected in an anergic response to tuberculin.

In dual infections there is a high frequency of extrapulmonary involvement often with concomitant pulmonary tuberculosis. The most frequent forms of extra-pulmonary disease are lymphadenitis and miliary disease, with increasing recognition of involvement of the bone marrow, genitourinary tract and central nervous system.

Infections due to atypical mycobacteria, such as *M. avium-intracellulare*, are uncommon in Africa. They are however a cause of disease in patients with AIDS, particularly in the United States. Most of the cases occur after other AIDS symptoms, and are attributed to exogenous infection.

Most AIDS patients with tuberculosis respond to standard antituberculosis drugs, although side-effects tend to be more frequent and the appropriate duration of treatment is not known. Cutaneous hypersensitivity reactions to thiacetazone are common, and can be fatal, in HIV seropositive patients.

Better methods for the identification of individuals with tuberculous infection, improvements in active case-finding, studies to assess the efficacy of tuberculous chemoprophylaxis in persons with HIV infection, development of vaccines other than BCG, and the development of improved and cheaper drugs for treatment are all priorities if the potential disease burden of tuberculosis interacting with HIV infection is to be controlled.

14
Leprosy

Mycobacterium leprae causes a chronic infection of skin, mucosae and peripheral nerves, the clinical effects of which depend on the immunological response of the host. It is an acid-alcohol-fast bacillus, related to *M. tuberculosis*, which can be cultured only in suckling mouse footpads or by inoculation of armadillos or mangabey monkeys. It is an obligate parasite of macrophages and the Schwann cells of peripheral nerves. The earliest sign of leprosy is a small number of hypopigmented skin plaques ('indeterminate leprosy'); in up to 90% of those affected a natural immunological cure occurs. 'Tuberculoid' leprosy is characterized by small numbers of hypopigmented anaesthetic skin plaques containing granulomas and small numbers of bacilli. 'Lepromatous' leprosy has multiple skin lesions containing many bacilli in abundant macrophages. 'Borderline' leprosy has features of both 'polar' types and may develop in either direction depending on the level of cell-mediated immunity, which is high in tuberculoid and low in lepromatous disease.

Susceptibility to infection, and the efficacy of the immune response to it, are determined by genetic factors, nutritional status, social factors such as housing, and intensity of duration of exposure to infective multi-bacillary cases, who spread the disease mainly by droplets from infected nasal mucosa. Transmission through the placenta, in breast milk and by insects is possible but unproven.

The clinical spectrum of leprosy is shown in the diagram on the following page.

ID leprosy skin macules are very few in number, with reduced pigment but normal sensation and sweating. They may persist for up to 2 years, but up to 90% heal completely. Lesions are commonly on the back, forearms, thighs, or face.

ID
Indeterminate

BB
Borderline

TT	BT	BL	LL
Tuberculoid	Borderline Tuberculoid	Borderline Lepromatous	Lepromatous

TT Leprosy has a few asymmetrical macules with slightly raised distinct edges, sensory loss and lack of sweating. In dark skins, the lesions are pale; in fair skins, slightly red. Thickening occurs of a few peripheral nerves asymmetrically. Biopsy shows epithelioid granulomas with giant cells and scanty bacilli.

In **BT leprosy** the skin lesions are more numerous and more peripheral nerves are involved.

In **BB leprosy** there are more skin lesions, often raised and ring-shaped, with normal or slightly reduced sensation, but with thickening of many peripheral nerves. **BL** cases have many small polymorphic shiny skin lesions.

In **LL leprosy** the skin lesions are numerous, widespread, symmetrical and may be macules, papules or nodules, with indistinct edges and a greasy appearance. Sensation in the lesions is usually normal, but peripheral nerve involvement is widespread, with generalized sensory and motor impairment.

Many areas of skin are liable to neuropathic damage because of loss of pain and temperature appreciation. The nasal mucosa is obviously involved. Corneal denervation leads to keratitis and iritis, and this is aggravated if facial nerve palsy is present. The eyebrows are lost. Neuropathic ulcers on the hands and feet develop with loss of digits, and bone loss also occurs in the nose. The testes and lymph nodes are damaged. Patients may present with painless burns or ulcers, which are often secondarily infected, with muscle weakness, nasal discharge, painful eyes or generalized systemic symptoms, including fever.

Of particular importance in the management of leprosy are the reaction states which occur:

1. **Type 1 ('Reversal' or 'upgrading') reaction.** This occurs in BT and BB, and some BL cases, usually after some weeks of treatment, but can occur in untreated cases. It results from increased cell-mediated immunity and causes inflammation

and swelling in existing skin lesions, which become red and painful, and a rapid onset of inflammation in affected peripheral nerves, resulting in pain and loss of function. The patient feels generally unwell with fever and joint pains.
2. **Type 2 (Erythema nodosum leprosum) reaction.** This occurs in up to 50% of LL cases, often if inadequately treated, as a result of excess immune complexes causing widespread vasculitis (Arthus reaction). New tender hot subcutaneous nodules develop, waxing and waning, and may become sterile pustules. Fever, iritis, nephritis, arthritis, orchitis and peripheral neuritis can occur to emphasize the multi-system nature of LL leprosy and of this reaction state in particular.
3. **'Downgrading' reaction.** This occurs in untreated or inadequately treated cases typically of BT, becoming BL, and even LL, with new lesions, more bacilli, and falling cell-mediated immunity. There is no increase in inflammation and no systemic symptoms.

The possible differential diagnoses of leprosy are summarized in Table 14.1.

The diagnosis of leprosy is primarily clinical, by examination of the skin and peripheral nerves in detail, noting especially pain sensation, sweating and motor function, as well as nerve thickening. Final proof rests on the demonstration of *M. leprae* in stained material from skin-slit smears from the edges of lesions or ear lobe, or smears from nasal mucosa. Classification within the spectrum is achieved by quantification of a **bacterial index** on a logarithmic scale (1+ is 1–10 bacilli in 100 fields, 6+ is 1000 bacilli in 1 field) and a **morphological index** is devised from the degree of stain uptake by bacilli. Biopsies of lesion edges or peripheral nerves are also stained to show bacilli. A skin test with lepromin will show a granulomatous nodule at one month (Mitsuda reaction) in TT and BT cases, but also in many who have healed ID lesions.

The treatment of multi-bacillary leprosy (LL, BL, BB, and BT cases with one or more positive smears) is with triple therapy:

1. rifampicin 600 mg monthly orally, supervised;
2. clofazimine 300 mg monthly orally, supervised and 50 mg daily unsupervised. Clofazimine causes diffuse dark red discoloration of the skin, with drying; patients who cannot accept this may be given ethionamide instead;
3. dapsone 100 mg daily orally, unsupervised.

Table 14.1 Differential diagnosis of leprosy

Differential diagnosis of leprosy
Infections
Onchocerciasis (skin and eyes)
Dermatophyte infections
Cutaneous leishmaniasis, esp. diffuse
Post kala-azar dermal leishmaniasis (PKDL)
Lupus vulgaris (TB)
Yaws

Other skin conditions
Vitiligo
Granuloma multiforme
Sarcoidosis of skin
Systemic lupus erythematosus
Lichen simplex
Lichen planus
Psoriasis
Kaposi's sarcoma
Seborrhoeic dermatitis
Neurofibromatosis
Skin metastases, e.g. of Hodgkin's disease
Keloid
Cauterization
Tribal scarification
Moxibustion
Peripheral neuropathy e.g. due to cassava

Treatment should be continued for at least 2 years and until all smears are negative (LL 5–10 years, BL 3–6 years, BB 2–3 years, BT 2 years).

Paucibacillary cases (ID, TT and smear-negative BT) should receive rifampicin 600 mg daily (unsupervised) and dapsone 100 mg daily (unsupervised) for 6 months, or until steroid treatment needed for Type 1 reaction is completed.

Reaction states should be treated as follows:

1. **Type 1 (reversal-upgrading).** Corticosteroids should be given urgently in a sufficient dose to control skin and nerve inflammation. Active neuritis may require the use of splints, and in a few cases surgical decompression of inflamed nerves is needed. Chemotherapy is continued unchanged.
2. **Type 2 (ENL)** may be treated with anti-inflammatory drugs (e.g. aspirin, thalidomide, chloroquine) but often steroids are

also needed. An increase in dose of clofazimine may be helpful. The other chemotherapy is given unchanged.
3. **Downgrading** reactions simply require adequate standard chemotherapy.

General care of leprosy patients is important, especially in LL disease. This includes good nutrition, splinting when neuritis is active, protection of anaesthetic areas, especially in the feet by shoes or sandals, and surgical treatment of ulcers, contractures and neuropathic joints. Indolent ulcers of the feet are common and difficult to heal.

Prevention of leprosy depends mainly on active case-finding, especially of LL (infectious) disease, by the education of primary health care workers and the general population, followed by effective treatment. Socio-economic improvement, especially of housing, may play a part. A new killed *M. leprae* vaccine is now under trial, and it is hoped that this will provide better protection than the limited benefit given by the use of BCG vaccine for tuberculosis. It remains true that in many societies a major social stigma attaches to leprosy, which is therefore concealed. One family member may seek treatment and then distribute the medicines received among the other infected relations. Leprosy is a common disease in many tropical countries, especially in West and Central Africa, Ethiopia, India, Myanmar, Nepal, the Pacific Islands, Madagascar, Brazil and Surinam.

15
Leptospirosis and Relapsing Fever

LEPTOSPIROSIS

Aetiology and epidemiology

Leptospirosis is probably the commonest infection of vertebrates transmitted to man. The genus *Leptospira* contains two species of aerobic Gram-negative spirochaetes: *L. biflexa* comprises aquatic saprophytic strains, whereas *L. interrogans* contains 202 pathogenic serovars (formerly termed serotypes) in 23 serogroups. The prevalence of individual serovars varies with geographical location.

As a rule, infected wild and domestic animals remain well, although they excrete leptospires in their urine and may become chronic excretors. Leptospires survive in moist environments outside the host but are destroyed by acidity and desiccation. Humans become infected by exposure to animal urine, blood or tissues, or to contaminated water. Man becomes infected when leptospires penetrate the mucous membranes of the eyes and nasopharynx, or skin abrasions, or following inhalation of infected material.

Leptospirosis is especially common in tropical countries with heavy rainfall and neutral or alkaline soil. Transmission is often seasonal, increasing in the rainy season when organisms deposited beside water are carried into rivers and streams as the water levels rise. Vocational and recreational activities which pose a risk include working in rice fields, fishing, farming, trapping, slaughtering or caring for animals, swimming, wading, rafting or boating in fresh water.

Clinical features

After entry organisms rapidly multiply and infect most tissues of the body. The incubation period is 7–12 days (range 2–26 days). Infection in man results in an illness which varies from a mild febrile condition to fulminant septicaemia with renal failure. Some cases are subclinical and pass unnoticed. The disease may follow a biphasic pattern; the first leptospiraemic phase resembles influenza, whereas the second is characterized by multisystem involvement, with the disappearance of leptospires from the blood, leptospiruria and a rising antibody titre.

Most patients present with sudden onset of fever, rigors, nausea, vomiting, conjunctival suffusion and headache. Severe myalgia may be localized to certain muscle groups, particularly the calf, lumbosacral spine or abdominal wall, or it may be generalized or associated with extreme cutaneous hyperaesthesia. Abdominal symptoms may be severe and when associated with diarrhoea may mimic gastroenteritis. Spontaneous recovery without specific treatment usually occurs within 2 weeks, but a few patients develop lymphocytic meningitis as a manifestation of the immunological response. In severe cases, the patient's general condition deteriorates over a period of about 7 days and cholestatic jaundice and renal failure develop. Adult respiratory distress syndrome, uveitis and intravascular coagulation are rare complications. About 10–20% of these patients die as a result of vascular collapse, massive haemorrhage, myocarditis or renal failure. This severe illness is more commonly, but not exclusively, due to infection with the *icterohaemorrhagiae* serovar.

Diagnosis

Early diagnosis requires a high index of suspicion. Leptospires can be isolated from blood, cerebrospinal fluid and urine, but the diagnosis is usually established by detecting specific serum antibodies. The complement fixation test (CFT) does not become positive until days 7–10 and peaks at around 3 weeks. Occasional non-specific reactions occur in hepatitis A, syphilis, mycoplasma and cytomegalovirus infection. The microscopic agglutination test does not become positive until day 6–9 and an IgM ELISA at 5–6 days after the onset of symptoms. Early antibiotic treatment, which needs to be given before serological confirmation is possible, can suppress antibody titres and low titres can persist for months or years after infection.

During the second phase of disease with signs of meningitis, examination of the CSF will reveal a lymphocytosis associated with modest increase in protein levels and normal blood glucose.

Treatment

Once leptospirosis is clinically suspected, adequate symptomatic, antibiotic and supportive treatment should be initiated. The main aim of antimicrobial therapy is to prevent complications, so it must be given early, i.e. within the first week of illness before serological confirmation is possible.

Benzyl penicillin 1.5 megaunits or ampicillin 1 g every 6 hours intravenously for 7 days should be given. Penicillin can induce a short-lived so-called 'MacKay-Dick' reaction, which is regarded as a sign of leptospiral lysis.

Doxycycline 100 mg orally twice daily for 7 days is an appropriate alternative in patients allergic to penicillin who are not too ill to take oral treatment. Erythromycin 500 mg every 6 hours intravenously is a suitable alternative to penicillin where parenteral administration is necessary.

Recent studies have shown that intravenous penicillin is better than placebo in severe and late leptospirosis.

Prevention and control

Rodent control around human habitation along with good animal husbandry practices combined with avoidance of potentially contaminated waters and soil are prerequisites for prevention and control. Those in contact with water likely to be infected should wear protective clothing and cover all cuts and abrasions with waterproof dressings. Large-scale vaccination of domestic animals with a high potency vaccine of a composition relevant to the local strains of the region can prevent both disease in animals and renal excretion of the organism. Human vaccines have been used with varied success in high risk groups but can also produce severe side-effects and are not routinely available.

Doxycyline 200 mg weekly may protect those at high risk for short periods.

RELAPSING FEVER

Louse-borne relapsing fever

Aetiology and epidemiology
Louse-borne relapsing fever is caused by the spirochaete *Borrelia recurrentis*. Man is the only mammalian host and the disease is transmitted from man to man by the body louse, *Pedicularis humanus* var. *corporis*, and by the head louse, *Pedicularis humanus* var. *capitis*. Louse-borne infection occurs in epidemics in areas of poverty, overcrowding and poor personal hygiene. Endemic foci exist in Africa (particularly the highlands of Ethiopia and Burundi), South America (the Peruvian Andes) and Asia (China and Vietnam). Lice become infected by feeding on blood from a person in the febrile phase of relapsing fever, when spirochaetes are present in the peripheral blood. There is no transovarial transmission within the louse population. The spirochaetes in the louse become infective after a period of 6 days. Man is not infected by the louse bite, but by crushing the louse and scratching the spirochaetes released from the louse through a break in the skin. Lice like to leave the body when there is a high fever, or when temperature drops due to death or exposure, thus favouring transmission. Other modes of transmission include transplacental infection and transfusion of infected blood.

The spirochaetes multiply and disseminate widely via the bloodstream. Circulating antibodies develop and clear borreliae from the blood. New antigenic variants emerge and give rise to the relapsing nature of the disease.

Clinical features
The incubation period is usually 4–8 days. Louse-borne relapsing fever is characterized by a primary attack of fever followed by up to four relapses. The illness begins abruptly with high fever, rigors, headache and myalgia, Nausea, vomiting, diarrhoea, abdominal pain, and cough and dyspnoea may be present early in the illness. Fever lasts on average for 5 days and is followed by an afebrile period of about a week. Fever then recurs, but is generally milder and shorter in duration than the initial episode. Findings include meningism, hepatosplenomegaly and a rash that may be macular, papular or petechial, and can be generalized or focal. There is conjunctival suffusion and subconjunctival haemorrhages may be present. Less common findings are jaun-

dice and tender lymphadenopathy. Complications include pneumonia, myocarditis (presenting as pulmonary oedema), nephritis, arthritis, neuropathy, iridocyclitis, meningoencephalitis, and severe bleeding due to thrombocytopenia, liver failure, and disseminated intravascular coagulation. Case mortality even with treatment is around 5%. Patients with louse-borne relapsing fever often have other intercurrent infections such as malaria, tuberculosis, salmonellosis and typhoid.

Diagnosis
Borreliae are usually found in thick blood films, stained with Wright's or Giemsa stains, or acridine orange, during a febrile episode. Dark ground microscopy can also be employed. Serological tests cross-react with other spirochaetes and are unreliable.

Treatment
Louse-borne relapsing fever is readily cured with a single oral dose of 500 mg of tetracycline or erythromycin. Treatment may induce a severe Jarisch-Herxheimer reaction which may prove fatal. The reaction is not prevented by pretreatment with steroids, but meptazinol diminishes the reaction when given in a dose of up to 500 mg by intravenous injection.

Prevention and control
Patients with relapsing fever are infectious until they have been thoroughly deloused. Heat sterilization of clothing kills lice eggs.

Tick-borne relapsing fever

Aetiology and epidemiology
A number of species of *Borrelia* including *B. duttoni* are causal organisms of tick-borne relapsing fever. Transmission to man is by the bite of an adult or nymph soft tick of the genus *Ornithodorus*. The tick remains infected for many years and transovarial transmission of borrelia to its offspring occurs.

Man is the only source of *B. duttoni* infection for *O. moubata*, the vector of disease in east, central and southern Africa. Elsewhere in north Africa, the eastern Mediterranean, central Asia and North and South America, tick-borne disease is a zoonosis and *Borrelia* species are found in rodents and other animals on which a variety of *Ornithodorus* ticks feed. Infection in man is accidental when exposure to ticks occurs in rodent habitats such as burrows, caves and infested buildings.

Clinical features
There is an incubation period of up to 14 days. The clinical course is similar to, though milder than, the louse-borne form. A primary attack may be followed by up to 11 relapses, occurring at intervals of 2 to 20 days. The borreliae of tick-borne relapsing fever are neurotropic and can give rise to lymphocytic meningitis, cranial nerve palsies and a variety of other central nervous system manifestations.

Diagnosis
Borreliae are present in the blood during febrile periods, but are fewer in number than in louse-borne disease. Organisms can be amplified by injection into rats or mice.

Treatment
Treatment is as for louse-borne disease. The Jarisch-Herxheimer reaction is not a complication of treatment.

Prevention and control
Tick-infested human habitations can be sprayed with acaricides. Personal protection includes the use of tick repellents and permethrin on clothing and bedding for persons with exposure in endemic foci. Antibiotic chemoprophylaxis with tetracycline may be used after exposure to a tick bite when the risk of acquiring the infection is high.

16
Acute Bacterial Meningitis

Bacterial meningitis is an acute and serious illness associated with significant morbidity and mortality. It is a common cause of illness in the tropics and makes a significant contribution to infant mortality. *Streptococcus pneumoniae* (pneumococcal meningitis) and *Haemophilus influenzae* are the most common causes of acute bacterial meningitis in the tropics, but *Neisseria meningitidis* (meningococcal meningitis) is the most common in the northern savannah belt of tropical Africa.

MENINGOCOCCAL MENINGITIS

Aetiology and epidemiology

In most areas of the tropics meningococcal infection is endemic; sporadic cases are seen from time to time but major outbreaks are unusual. In sub-Saharan Africa, however, meningococcal meningitis epidemics have been documented to recur in 8 to 12 year cycles during the dry season. In this 'meningitis belt' between the Sahara in the north and the equatorial forest in the south there are some 10 000 cases of meningitis each epidemic year with an average case mortality of around 12%.

Transmission is by droplet spread from person to person. Asymptomatic nasopharyngeal infections are more frequent than clinical disease, and carriers rather than patients are the usual source of new infections. Close contact favours the spread of meningococci and the immediate contacts of a patient are at high risk of infection. During epidemics attack rates for meningococcal disease are highest among the least privileged sections of the community. In the African 'meningitis belt' there is an upsurge of cases during the months of January through to March. During this period the climate is dry and the nights particularly cold. The dry climatic conditions predispose to dry nasopharyngeal mucous membranes, reducing their efficiency as a barrier to infection, whilst the cold nights bring people into closer proximity huddled together indoors, giving ideal conditions for disease transmission.

Neisseria meningitidis has been classified into eight main serogroups based on the differences in capsular polysaccharides. Cases of meningococcal meningitis are usually caused by organisms belonging to serogroups A, B, C and W135. There are considerable geographical variations in the distribution of serogroups responsible for disease. Whilst most cases in the United States and Europe are caused by groups B and C, most African epidemics are caused by group A meningococci, although outbreaks of group C disease have been reported in West Africa. Epidemics of group A meningococcal meningitis have recently occurred outside the 'meningitis belt' (in Kenya and Tanzania in 1989 and in Uganda in 1990), and also in Nepal and Saudi Arabia.

Clinical features

Clinical infection occurs when nasopharyngeal carriage of meningococci gives rise to a bacteraemia. Bacteraemia is probably the primary event in all forms of infection, though it has been suggested that the meninges might be infected by direct spread through the cribriform plate. Most patients with a systemic meningococcal infection present with meningitis, a minority present with acute meningococcal septicaemia, and a few have features of both clinical syndromes.

Acute meningococcaemia is usually of swift onset and is often rapidly fulminating. Onset is usually with fever and tachycardia with the early appearance of cutaneous and conjunctival petechiae which progress to areas of ecchymoses which may become confluent. Diarrhoea is sometimes an early feature of the disease. The patient becomes drowsy and confused, tachypnoeic, tachycardic and profoundly hypotensive. Patients with meningococcaemia may die a matter of hours after the initial onset of symptoms from irreversible peripheral circulatory collapse, haemorrhage and myocarditis with cardiac arrhythmias and failure.

Meningococcaemia may follow a more benign course with low grade fever and the appearance of scattered petechiae. This clinical picture of blood culture positive but relatively asymptomatic meningococcal disease is seen most frequently at the end of an epidemic period in African patients.

The onset of meningococcal meningitis is often more gradual and gives rise to the classic symptoms and signs of bacterial meningitis.

Diagnosis

Meningococcaemia should be considered in the differential diagnosis of any patient with a fever and petechial rash, along with a consideration of other Gram-negative bacteraemias, rickettsial diseases and dengue.

Acute meningococcal meningitis, in the absence of a rash, cannot be reliably distinguished from other forms of bacterial meningitis. Cerebrospinal fluid examination will reveal the typical cytological and biochemical characteristics of a bacterial meningitis. Meningococci can be demonstrated microscopically in up to 80% of untreated cases. Detection of meningococcal capsular polysaccharide antigen in the CSF is highly specific.

Treatment

Crystalline penicillin is the antibiotic of choice for the treatment of meningococcal meningitis. Parenteral administration of penicillin in the appropriate dose regimen for 5 days is sufficient total treatment. Longer courses of treatment are not necessary. If for any reason the patient cannot be given penicillin, then chloramphenicol is an effective substitute, and has the advantage that oral therapy can be started as soon as a patient is conscious. Concern, however, because of the occasional case of aplastic anaemia following chloramphenicol, limits its more widespread use. Sulphonamides should not be used because of increasingly widespread resistance of meningococci to this antibiotic. There is no role for combination antibiotic therapy.

In hot climates patients with meningitis who are febrile, may have stopped drinking and may well have been vomiting, are often markedly dehydrated and will require urgent rehydration.

When major outbreaks of meningococcal meningitis occur routine health facilities may be overwhelmed. It may be necessary to establish temporary treatment centres providing treatment with a single injection of long-acting antibiotic. An oily injection of chloramphenicol in the appropriate dose can be very effective for meningococcal meningitis, but not that due to *Haemophilus influenzae* type b or the pneumococcus.

Dexamethasone has recently been advocated for early use in the treatment of meningococcal meningitis, in combination with antibiotic treatment. It has been demonstrated to block and decrease the toxic effects of the interleukins and tumour necrosis factor (TNF) which occur with lysis of bacterial cell walls. Currently investigation of the role of non-steroidal anti-inflammatory agents and therapeutic intervention with monoclonal antibodies such as interleukin and TNF blocking agents is being undertaken.

Acute meningococcaemia is a medical emergency requiring early parenteral treatment with penicillin and a wide variety of supportive measures including the careful monitoring of fluid balance, acid-base status, central venous pressure and blood pressure. Hypotensive shock is a frequent complication of acute meningococcaemia and an important cause of death. Bleeding, associated with disseminated intravascular coagulation, may be severe and require treatment with fresh blood. Large doses of dexamethasone given as early as possible appear to improve the considerable morbidity and mortality of this disease.

A proportion of patients with acute meningococcaemia or meningitis develop arthritis, pericarditis or cutaneous vasculitis some 5 to 10 days after the onset of their illness. These complications are due to the formation of immune complexes and do not necessitate the prolongation of antibiotic treatment and should be treated symptomatically.

Prevention and control

When the infection is sporadic attention should be concentrated on close contacts of patients and prevention and control measures depend upon chemoprophylaxis and vaccination.

Sulphonamide-resistant meningococci are widespread in Africa and preclude its generalized use as a chemoprophylactic agent. Rifampicin is effective in eliminating meningococci from the nasopharynx, but is expensive and its widespread use may lead to the emergence of rifampicin-resistant meningococci or, in countries where tuberculosis and leprosy are prevalent, rifampicin resistance in these mycobacteria. A full course of parenteral penicillin may be considered for a very close contact of the patient as a means of treating possible early disease. Penicillin will not however eliminate nasopharyngeal carriage of the organism.

Vaccines are available against groups A, C, W135 and Y. The capsular polysaccharide of the group B meningococcus is poorly immunogenic and a candidate vaccine for this group is not yet available. Vaccination has proved successful in reducing infection (but not carriage) rates in parts of Africa. Existing vaccines are poorly immunogenic in children under 2 years of age. Capsular polysaccharide antigens fail, at this age, to induce a T cell response with the result that antibody levels are poor and show no memory response. In older persons good antibody levels are not achieved for some 10 to 14 days and vaccination cannot therefore substitute for chemoprophylaxis in controlling infection in household contacts. It has been suggested that vaccination might be considered for contacts of cases with group A or C infections in addition to chemoprophylaxis, in order to protect against the longer-term increased risk of infection.

If an outbreak of disease is caused by a meningococcus belonging to a serogroup for which a vaccine is available, an early mass immunization programme should be mounted. Epidemiological studies will indicate the age and geographical distribution of persons requiring vaccination. If it is known that a certain epidemic strain is sensitive to sulphonamides then widespread sulphonamide chemoprophylaxis can be used in conjunction with a vaccination campaign.

During African epidemics attempts have been made to reduce transmission by encouraging people to sleep out of doors and by banning markets and festivals, but evidence as to the effectiveness of these interventions is unconvincing.

HAEMOPHILUS INFLUENZAE MENINGITIS

Aetiology and epidemiology

Worldwide most cases of haemophilus meningitis are due to a single serotype – type b. Very high rates of disease are seen in Australian aboriginals and native Americans – Eskimos and Indians. There are few data available from developing countries but those available indicate that the incidence is high. Further, the morbidity and mortality of meningitis may be significantly greater in developing countries than in developed countries.

Clinical features

Like the meningococcus, *Haemophilus influenzae* type b (Hib) colonizes the nasopharynx. Peak carriage occurs in children. The average age of those developing disease is much younger than those developing meningococcal disease and some 60% of Hib disease in developing countries occurs in infants aged less than 12 months. The commonest clinical syndrome is meningitis, but bacteraemia, epiglottitis, arthritis, cellulitis and other acute pyogenic infections occur.

Meningitis due to *H. influenzae* cannot be distinguished with certainty on clinical grounds from that due to other bacteria. Case fatality rates from meningitis vary from less than 5% (USA) to 30% (Papua New Guinea).

Diagnosis

The cytology and chemistry of the cerebrospinal fluid (CSF) fails to distinguish haemophilus meningitis from other bacterial causes. Organisms may be identified microscopically, typed with antiserum, and cultured from CSF and blood.

Treatment

The impact of antibiotics in preventing death from invasive *H. influenzae* is limited by economic constraints and the emergence of drug-resistant strains. There has been an emergence and worldwide increase in frequency of ampicillin resistance. Resistance to chloramphenicol is as yet uncommon although there have been reports of *H. influenzae* strains resistant to both ampicillin and chloramphenicol. Chloramphenicol is still the drug of choice. At first 500 mg (children 25 mg/kg) should be given intravenously and then orally 6-hourly for 10 days.

Prevention and control

Bacterial capsular polysaccharides are poor immunogens, especially in children less than 2 years old where the brunt of infection falls. However, new type b polysaccharide-protein conjugate vaccines are immunogenic in infants as young as 2 months of age. But, for developing countries, more complete data defining the populations at risk, the immunogenicity of candidate vaccines in different ethnic groups, and the serotypes of the infecting organisms will be needed before successful cost-effective vaccination strategies can be devised and implemented.

PNEUMOCOCCAL MENINGITIS

Meningitis due to *Streptococcus pneumoniae* is the commonest cause of bacterial meningitis in children with sickle cell disease or in patients who have had a splenectomy. The clinical picture and CSF findings are similar to other forms of bacterial meningitis.

Pneumococcal meningitis can result as a complication of bacteraemic pneumonia or secondary to such infections as mastoiditis and sinusitis, or may follow damage to the base of the skull. But in up to 40% of cases no obvious primary focus is found. The disease is seen in all age groups, and the mortality in developing countries is around 50%, being highest in infants and the elderly. Significant neurological sequelae are encountered in about 10–20% of survivors.

Penicillin G remains the antibiotic of choice in patients with pneumococcal meningitis. Crystalline penicillin 2.4 g (children 600 mg to 1.2 g) should be given 6 hourly for 14 days. For patients who are known to be allergic to penicillin, chloramphenicol is an effective alternative and penetrates well into the CSF. An increasing number of pneumococcal infections are being reported as being resistant to penicillin treatment. In such cases a change to chloramphenicol or a third-generation cephalosporin, based on *in vitro* sensitivities where available, should be made.

BACTERIAL MENINGITIS – ORGANISM NOT IDENTIFIED

The causative organism of meningitis is not always identified. Identification is often particularly difficult in patients who have received partial antibiotic treatment. Lumbar puncture is best avoided if there is severe depression of consciousness or if there are fits, focal neurological signs or papilloedema – all rare events in meningitis. In this situation chloramphenicol is the antibiotic treatment of choice. It is effective against *H. influenzae* and both meningococcus and pneumococcus and penetrates well into the CSF. It should not be used in neonates and infants unless serum concentrations can be closely monitored because of the risk of severe toxicity and 'grey baby' syndrome. Single-dose treatment with a long-acting chloramphenicol preparation (Tifomycine) during meningitis epidemics has been effective, provided there is no extrameningeal focus of infection.

17
Enteric Fever

Enteric fever is caused by *Salmonella typhi* and *S. paratyphi* A and B, which are Gram-negative bacteria causing exclusively human infections, characterized initially by fever. The bacteria are transmitted by ingestion of food or water contaminated by faeces or urine of active cases of disease or healthy carriers of the infections.

S. typhi has three antigens:

1. cell wall lipopolysaccharide O;
2. heat-labile polysaccharide virulence antigen of outer capsule Vi;
3. flagella H.

Bacteria invade intestinal lymphoid tissue, multiply in macrophages, and are disseminated by blood to the liver, spleen and bone marrow, where the release of cytokines (interleukin 1, tumour necrosis factor) is induced, and monocytes proliferate. Bacteraemia is then followed by secondary invasion of the small intestine, leading to ileitis with diarrhoea and the possibility of perforation of and haemorrhage from inflamed Peyer's patches. Infection of the gallbladder occurs during this phase and may cause acute cholecystitis and subsequently become the source of chronic excretion of the organisms.

The clinical illness of typhoid (enteric) fever classically begins with a progressive onset of fever with chills (but no rigors), headache and abdominal distension and discomfort with constipation, although in epidemic disease from a single source patients may present with acute diarrhoea and vomiting with headache and meningism. After several days of fever a pale red macular rash may appear on the trunk ('rose spots') and splenomegaly is usually evident. Epistaxis and deafness may occur. In at least 10%

of cases there is evidence of involvement of the central nervous system, with delirium, acute psychosis, cerebellar signs, a midbrain syndrome or fits in children. A pulse rate elevation lower than that expected from the height of the fever ('relative bradycardia') is a classical feature but may be absent. From the second week of fever onwards the patient becomes toxic and cachectic, with the risk of intestinal perforation and haemorrhage, due to enteritis. Untreated mortality is 10–15% mostly in small children. With treatment in good facilities this should be reduced below 1%.

Possible complications of typhoid fever include pneumonia, myocarditis, osteomyelitis, arthritis, and mastitis. The illness may relapse after apparent cure by antibiotic therapy, a similar but milder illness appearing 7 to 14 days after defervescence in 5 to 10% of those treated with chloramphenicol.

Diagnosis is best made by culture of the organism from:

1. blood (whole or clotted);
2. stool (from the 2nd week);
3. urine (from the 2nd week);
4. bone marrow – especially useful if some antibiotic treatment has been given;
5. duodenal juice – by aspiration or Enterotest string;
6. 'rose spot' biopsy.

The standard serological test (Widal) is unreliable but a four-fold rise in titre against O antigen between two specimens is diagnostic. Antibody to H antigen is raised in those previously immunized, but negative in up to 30% of proven cases.

Proven cases almost always have a significant leukopenia (granulopenia).

The differential diagnosis includes malaria, typhus, viral hepatitis, amoebic liver abscess, other infective causes of enteritis, infectious mononucleosis, brucellosis, Q fever and bacterial endocarditis.

Treatment of typhoid fever may be with:

1. chloramphenicol 60 mg/kg/day, divided 6-hourly, orally or intravenously, for 3–4 days, then 30 mg/kg/day for 6–10 days;
2. cotrimoxazole, 2 tablets twice daily for 14 days;
3. amoxycillin (1 g q.i.d. for 14 days) or ampicillin.

Resistance to any or all of these antibiotics is now common in many tropical countries, but management depends on availability and cost of alternatives. Ciprofloxacin 500 mg b.d. orally for 10 days is an effective treatment.

Cases of typhoid fever require careful nursing, with attention to fluid balance, blood transfusion if intestinal haemorrhage occurs, and surgical treatment of intestinal perforation. Severely toxic patients benefit from the addition of corticosteroid treatment, e.g. dexamethasone. Relapses should be treated as for the first attack. Chronic intestinal excretion can be treated with amoxycillin with periodical or prolonged courses of cotrimoxazole or norfloxacin; occasionally cholecystectomy may be needed.

Typhoid fever is common in all tropical countries, flourishing where sanitation and food hygiene are poor. Control in communities depends on improved sanitation and water treatment and control of restaurants and food handlers. Personal protection can be enhanced by vaccines:

1. monovalent killed *S. typhi* 0.5 ml s.c. with 0.1 ml i.d. 4 weeks later, boosted as needed at intervals of 3 years;
2. live attenuated oral Ty 21a – in 3 to 4 doses;
3. modified Vi antigen vaccine.

18

Tetanus

Tetanus is caused by *Clostridium tetani*, a spore-forming Gram-positive anaerobic bacillus, which is resistant to boiling and many antiseptics but is killed in an autoclave after 15 minutes. It is present in the faeces of many animals, especially bovines and horses, and infects the soil in all countries where cultivation of the land is widespread. Spores enter the skin through puncture wounds or lacerations, through the umbilical stump of neonates, through snake and animal bites and, less commonly, through *Dracunculus* ulcers and chronic suppurative otitis media, and in puerperal sepsis and induced abortions. Culture of the bacillus from contaminated wounds may be difficult because many other organisms also multiply.

Cl. tetani forms an exotoxin, tetanospasmin, which passes up the axons of motor neurones to the nerve cell body, and is delivered by blood to other neuro-muscular junctions. The toxin blocks inhibitory input from the brain stem by preventing GABA release, with the clinical effects of increased resting muscle tone and severe reflex muscle spasms.

The incubation period of clinical tetanus varies from a few days to several weeks; the longer the interval, the better the final prognosis. The entry wound may be healed or inapparent. The earliest symptom is a spasm of the masseter muscles, causing trismus; muscle spasm then spreads to the neck, back, abdomen and limbs, causing opisthotonos and clenching of the fists. Spasms may be induced by touch, noise or bright light and may last for several minutes, with compromise to respiration. Newborn babies infected through the umbilicus usually present aged 6 to 10 days with feeding difficulties, generalized spasms, and an infected umbilical stump, and quickly become dehydrated and exhausted. Most patients with tetanus have autonomic nervous dysfunction, resulting in lability of temperature and blood pressure, excessive sweating and cardiac dysrhythmias.

The diagnosis of tetanus is clinical; it should be distinguished from poisoning by strychnine and organophosphates, from phenothiazine dystonia and from status epilepticus, in infants from meningitis, encephalitis and hypocalcaemic tetany, and from the trismus caused by local jaw or mouth disease, including diphtheria.

On a diagnosis of tetanus being made, 3000 units of human tetanus immunoglobulin should be given i.m. An infected wound should be debrided, and antibiotic treatment started with parenteral crystalline penicillin. Mild spasms may be controllable with diazepam but severe cases require curarization and ventilation, often for many days. A quiet dark side-room should be used for nursing such patients. Parenteral nutrition should be given if possible. Neonatal tetanus is particularly difficult to treat and has a high mortality (50 to 80%), since injections and feeding induce severe spasms. Intrarectal paraldehyde or phenobarbitone can be employed. These infants are particularly at risk from hypothermia.

In developed countries, 70% of cases of tetanus occur over the age of 50 years, to individuals who have never been immunized or whose immunity has declined. Accidents while gardening are an important source of risk. In developing countries 70% of cases occur under the age of 10 years, complicating compound fractures and contaminated wounds or in neonates, there being an estimated 800 000 neonatal deaths annually from this cause worldwide.

The ideal preventive method for tetanus is to immunize the entire population with tetanus toxoid; this is usually given with diphtheria and pertussis vaccines in infancy and boosted at 1 and 5 years. Individuals subsequently suffering contaminated wounds should receive two boosting doses of toxoid and 250 units of tetanus immunoglobulin i.m.

The prevention of neonatal tetanus depends on the immunization of mothers with two doses of toxoid during pregnancy and on the education of mothers, midwives and traditional birth attendants in safe delivery practices, in particular by discouraging the application of animal dung or butter to the umbilical stump.

19
Sexually Transmitted Diseases

Sexually transmitted diseases (STDs) are an important cause of morbidity in both adults and infants born to infected mothers. In many health services in the developing world about 10% of all consultations are for an STD related problem, and in antenatal clinics up to 20% of women may have an undiagnosed STD.

Causes for concern are the increasing incidence of STDs worldwide, worsening antibiotic resistance patterns, and the recognition that STDs, and in particular genital ulcer disease, facilitate transmission of human immunodeficiency virus (HIV).

High rates of infertility, pelvic inflammatory disease and ectopic pregnancies are considered mainly to be a consequence of STDs.

Bacteria which cause STDs vary in their sensitivity to different antibiotics from area to area. This is partly because of the extent to which different antibiotics have been used in different countries, and partly due to the widespread problems of incomplete treatment and self treatment, which encourage the emergence of resistant strains. Specific treatment protocols should be worked out locally. Treatment schedules and alternatives given below are those recommended by the World Health Organization in 1989.

This chapter does not set out to supply a comprehensive and detailed description of STDs but rather to provide a brief and practical guide to their diagnosis and treatment in the setting of the developing world.

GENITAL ULCER DISEASE

The commonest sexually transmitted causes of genital ulceration are chancroid, primary syphilis, herpes simplex, lymphogranuloma venereum (LGV), granuloma inguinale and scabies. In some 25% of patients with genital ulcers no specific cause can be found. Diagnostic facilities may be less than ideal and a good clinical diagnosis based on a knowledge of the local epidemiology of genital ulcer disease and a careful history and examination are often required.

Chancroid is the commonest cause of genital ulceration in South-east Asia and Africa. Granuloma inguinale is more commonly seen in India and Papua New Guinea.

There are four questions to ask when a patient presents with genital ulcer disease:

1. Is the ulcer single or multiple?
2. What is the appearance of the lesion?
3. Is it painful?
4. Is there regional adenopathy and if so are the nodes painful?

Chancroid

Chancroid is caused by the bacillus *Haemophilus ducreyi* and has an incubation period of 1 to 15 days. It accounts for up to 60% of genital ulcers in parts of Africa.

Chancroid can cause either single or multiple ulcers, which may be very painful. The ulcers are usually irregular and necrotic and have a purulent base. The ulcers are soft, as opposed to indurated, and commonly bleed on contact. Regional lymphadenopathy is often unilateral and occurs in some two thirds of cases. Infected lymph nodes are painful and may enlarge to form a single mass or bubo. The bubo may rupture, characteristically through a single sinus, and cause extensive ulceration and local tissue damage, particularly if it becomes secondarily infected with anaerobic bacteria.

A Gram stain of the pus from the floor of the ulcer will on occasion demonstrate the Gram-negative bacillus.

Lesions should be kept clean and dry. Recommended treatment are:

1. Ceftriaxone 250 mg intramuscular injection as a single dose; or
2. Cotrimoxazole (trimethoprim 80 mg + sulphamethoxazole 400 mg) two tablets by mouth twice a day for 7 days; or
3. Erythromycin 500 mg orally three times daily for 7 days.

Treatment should be repeated for a further 7 days if the ulcers have not healed in one week. In patients with AIDS these regimens are often not effective.

Syphilis

Syphilis is caused by the spiral-shaped bacterium *Treponema pallidum* and has an incubation period of 9 to 90 days. In parts of Africa about 20% of genital ulcers are due to primary syphilis.

A single, indurated, painless ulcer or chancre is characteristic of syphilis. The base of the ulcer is clean and does not bleed easily. Painless lymph node enlargement may be present in both groins. The chancre persists for 2 to 5 weeks and then heals, even without treatment. Without treatment the disease becomes latent and may in the future develop into secondary and tertiary disease. In a female, the chancre of syphilis may be present on the vulva, the perineum, inside the vagina, or on the cervix, and because it is painless is often missed.

Treponema pallidum cannot be seen with the light microscope but requires the use of dark ground microscopy. Diagnosis is usually confirmed by serological methods.

Tests using non-treponemal antigens (VDRL, WR, Kahn, RPR) are quick and inexpensive and are the tests most commonly available in the developing world. They have a low specificity. They become positive some 5 weeks after infection and remain so for a considerable time, even after adequate treatment. The more specific tests (TPHA, FTA) are expensive and less widely available. They become positive about 3 weeks after infection and remain so throughout life despite adequate treatment.

The treatment for primary, secondary or latent syphilis of less than 2 years duration takes the following forms:

1. Benzathine benzyl penicillin G 2.4 million units in a single dose by intramuscular injection. Because of the large volume, the dose is usually given as two injections at separate sites;
2. Aqueous procaine penicillin G 1.2 million units daily by intramuscular injection for 10 days; or (for patients allergic to penicillin, and not pregnant);
3. Tetracycline 500 mg four times daily for 15 days;
4. Doxycycline 100 mg orally twice daily for 15 days.

Treatment for late and congenital syphilis is beyond the scope of this chapter and the reader is referred to the World Health Organization STD Treatment Strategies (see Bibliography).

Lymphogranuloma venereum

Lymphogranuloma venereum (LGV) is caused by *Chlamydia trachomatis* (L1, L2, L3 strains) and has an incubation period of 7 to 28 days. The initial lesion is a single small papule or vesicle, which may ulcerate, and is non-indurated and painless. This lesion often goes unrecognized. Infection of the local lymph nodes gives rise to initially firm, discrete and tender adenopathy. Nodes later become matted and may resolve or progress to softening and suppuration with local lymphoedema. The swelling usually has several centres and, in contrast to chancroid, gives rise to a multilocular bubo. The patient is often systemically ill with fevers and chills. The inguinal ligament may appear as a groove through the mass of matted nodes. If not treated at this stage the nodes are destroyed and lymphoedema of the penis or vulva may develop into permanent elephantiasis with gross distortion of the genitalia.

In women the pelvic nodes may be affected and cause symptoms and signs similar to pelvic inflammatory disease. LGV may give rise to a distal procto-colitis which untreated can lead to rectal strictures or a recto-vaginal fistula.

There is no simple laboratory confirmatory test for LGV. Treatment is with any of the following:

Doxycycline 100 mg orally twice daily for 14 days;
Tetracycline 500 mg orally four times daily for 14 days;
Erythromycin 500 mg orally four times daily for 14 days;
Sulphadiazine 1 g four times daily for 14 days.

Known contacts of the index case should also receive treatment. If the bubo is large and fluctuant it should be aspirated through healthy skin using a large bore needle. The bubo should not be incised and drained as this will delay healing.

Genital herpes

Genital infection with the *Herpes simplex* virus gives rise, after an incubation period of 2 to 7 days, to multiple, small vesicles which ulcerate to form multiple, non-indurated, painful lesions which may coalesce to form large areas of ulceration. These lesions heal in about 3 weeks, but repeated attacks may occur. Pain and tenderness is more often experienced in the initial attack than in recurrences. Moderately painful and tender inguinal adenopathy occurs in up to 50% of cases of initial infection.

In women the cervix is the commonest site of infection and may be asymptomatic. If a woman has evidence of genital herpes at the time of childbirth then there is a considerable risk of neonatal herpes infection from vaginal delivery and where possible a caesarian section is indicated.

There is no simple test to aid the diagnosis of genital herpes.

Drug treatment with acyclovir is expensive and often not available. Patients should be advised to keep lesions clean and dry and to avoid sexual intercourse during an attack.

Treatment of the primary attack with acyclovir 200 mg orally five times daily for 7 days reduces the formation of new lesions, the duration of pain, and time to healing. It probably has no influence on the development of recurrent disease. About half of the patients with genital herpes will develop recurrent disease. The lesions are less painful than the primary lesions and usually heal within 5 to 7 days.

Granuloma inguinale

Granuloma inguinale is caused by *Calymmatobacterium granulomatis* and has an incubation period of 7 to 90 days. The primary lesion starts as an indurated painless papule which progresses to form a beefy granulomatous ulcer which is well-defined and has a raised, rolled edge. The lesions are usually painless unless secondary infection is present. They bleed readily on contact. The inguinal nodes are not involved unless there is secondary infection. Subcutaneous granulomata may occur in the inguinal region and be mistaken for lymph nodes. These granulomata may develop into abscesses and rupture resulting in ulceration. Untreated these lesions spread and cause widespread tissue destruction. Healing leads to intense fibrosis and further anatomical distortion. Metastatic spread of the lesions and neoplastic change has been reported.

A stained smear taken from the edge of a granulomatous lesion may demonstrate the presence of Gram-negative rods with bipolar staining (Donovan bodies).

Treatment may follow one of the following regimens:

1. Trimethoprim (80 mg)/sulphamethoxazole (400 mg), two tablets orally twice daily for 14 days;
2. Tetracycline 500 mg orally four times daily for 14 days;
3. Chloramphenicol 500 mg orally four times daily for 21 days;
4. Gentamicin 1 mg/kg intramuscularly three times daily for 21 days.

Scabies

Scabies can lead to genital ulceration and this is often seen in association with scabetic lesions of the scrotum and thighs along with those of the trunk and extremities. Scabies is a cause of genital sores in children.

In **all** cases of genital ulcer disease the patient must be asked to refrain from sexual intercourse until the infection is cured. If the patient is unable to comply with this request then they should be encouraged to use, and where necessary instructed how to use, a condom.

The patient's sexual contacts where possible should be seen, receive sympathetic counselling, and treated where appropriate.

URETHRAL DISCHARGE IN MALES

Urethral discharge is the commonest presenting symptom in men in most STD clinics and generally denotes sexually acquired urethritis. Urethral discharge is either gonococcal, due to *Neisseria gonorrhoeae*, or non-gonococcal (NGU). *Chlamydia trachomatis* accounts for about 50% of all cases of non-gonococcal urethritis; some 30% are of undetermined aetiology, and *Trichomonas vaginalis, Ureaplasma urealyticum, Candida albicans* and *Herpes simplex* account for many of the rest.

Gonorrhoea has an incubation period of 2 to 5 days and gives rise to symptomatic infection in more than 95% of those infected. Symptoms are those of dysuria associated with profuse, thick, purulent or mucopurulent urethral discharge. Non-gonococcal urethritis has an incubation period of some 5 to 20 days and gives rise to mild to moderate dysuria and a thin, mucoid to mucopurulent discharge.

Management of urethral discharge depends on whether or not microscopy is available and on the skill of the microscopist. When a Gram-stained urethral smear shows Gram-negative bean-shaped intracellular diplococci, a presumptive diagnosis of gonorrhoea is made. When diplococci are not seen but more than five polymorphonuclear leukocytes are present per high-powered field, then a diagnosis of non-gonococcal urethritis is made.

Penicillinase-producing *N. gonorrhoea* account for roughly 50% of all cases of gonorrhoea. Ideally, therefore, facilities for culture and sensitivity testing of the organism are required for treatment to be optimized. Without this facility treatment must be given on the basis of local knowledge of the organism and its response to treatment.

Recommended treatment for uncomplicated gonorrhoea in both men and women can take one of the following forms:

1. Ceftriaxone 250 mg by intramuscular injection as a single dose (or equivalent alternative third generation cephalosporin);
2. Ciprofloxacin 500 mg as a single oral dose (contraindicated in children and pregnancy);
3. Spectinomycin 2 g by intramuscular injection as a single dose.

Possibly useful in some areas where the gonococcus remains sensitive are:

4. Amoxycillin 3 g orally plus probenicid 1 g orally as a single dose; or
5. Aqueous procaine penicillin G 4.8 million units by intramuscular injection plus probenicid 1 g orally.

Treatment of uncomplicated non-gonococcal urethritis and chlamydial infection is with:

6. Doxycyline 100 mg orally twice daily for 7 days;
7. Tetracycline 500 mg orally four times daily for 10 days;
8. Erythromycin 500 mg orally four times daily for 7 days.

All patients should be reviewed two weeks after completion of treatment. Patients treated for gonorrhoea may have evidence of non-gonococcal urethritis, having had a double infection, the non-gonococcal component of which was masked by the symptoms of gonorrhoea. These patients, along with those with evidence of persistent gonorrhoea, will require further treatment.

Sexual contacts of cases should be examined and if possible investigated. Treatment may need to be given on an empirical basis. Treatment of symptomatic cases may also require this approach when diagnostic facilities are not available. It may be desirable to treat all such cases initially for gonorrhoea, followed by a course of treatment for NGU.

VAGINAL DISCHARGE

Vaginal discharge may be unrelated to STDs. *Candida albicans* is a common cause of vaginitis and may present with vulval irritation and soreness, watery white or creamy vaginal discharge, external dysuria and dyspareunia. Examination will confirm the presence of a white discharge and usually reveals cheesy plaques adherent to the vaginal wall and vulva. Treatment is with intravaginal nystatin pessaries nightly for 14 nights or clotrimazole or miconazole 100 mg intravaginally nightly for seven nights. Nystatin cream can be applied for vulvitis. The male sexual partner requires treatment if the woman is experiencing recurrent infection or if the male has candidal balanitis.

Of the STD causes of vaginal discharge gonorrhoea, *Trichomonas vaginalis* and *C.trachomatis* are important causes.

Diagnosis based on clinical presentation is often inaccurate. A full screening of a patient with vaginal discharge should include a history of menstruation, contraception, antibiotic usage, sexual partners and symptoms, together with a careful examination of the external genitalia, vagina and cervix. Where laboratory facilities are available the appropriate microbiological investigations should be undertaken. Rough guidelines for the management of cases of vaginal discharge in the absence of laboratory confirmation are as follows:

1. If the discharge is white and there is evidence of white plaques of material adherent to the genital tract, then treatment should be given for candidiasis.
2. If the discharge is profuse and frothy treat for trichomonas. Metronidazole 2 g in a single oral dose should be given to both patient and sexual partner. Metronidazole is contraindicated in the first trimester of pregnancy. In this situation clotrimazole 100 mg intravaginally each night for seven nights may produce symptomatic relief and some cures.
3. If the discharge has a strong, fishy smell, treat for bacterial vaginosis with either:
   i. Metronidazole 500 g orally twice daily or 250 mg orally three times daily for 7 days; or
   ii. Metronidazole 2 g orally as a single dose, repeated after 48 hours.
4. If discharge is seen from the cervix, treat for both gonorrhoea and chlamydia.
5. If vaginal discharge is accompanied by lower abdominal pain and tenderness, treat for pelvic inflammatory disease.

PELVIC INFLAMMATORY DISEASE

If gonococcal or chlamydial infection in females is not treated early and effectively, it may spread to the pelvic organs and cause pelvic inflammatory disease (PID). The presenting symptoms include vaginal discharge, lower abdominal pain and tenderness, fever, menstrual disturbances, deep dyspareunia and backache.

On abdominal examination there is pelvic tenderness and on vaginal examination there may be a tender pelvic mass and cervical excitation tenderness. The differential diagnosis includes ectopic pregnancy, appendicitis and cystitis, as well as ovarian causes.

Recommended treatment is: Single dose treatment for gonorrhoea; plus tetracycline 500 mg orally four times daily for 10 days; plus metronidazole 500 mg three times daily for 10 days.

The patient's partner should be investigated and treated as appropriate.

OPHTHALMIA NEONATORUM

Over 40% of babies born to mothers with gonorrhoea acquire gonococcal conjunctivitis. Some 2 to 5 days after delivery, the eye becomes red and swollen, with profuse purulent discharge. Ophthalmia neonatorum may also develop in 35 to 50% of babies born to mothers with genital tract *C. trachomatis* infection. The incubation period for chlamydial conjunctivitis is 5 to 14 days; it is usually less severe than gonococcal disease.

The condition may be prevented by disinfection of the child's eyes at birth and the use of tetracycline or erythromycin eye ointment prophylactically.

A Gram-stained smear of conjunctival exudate will help differentiate between gonococcal and non-gonococcal disease. Mixed infections may occur.

Treatment should first be directed to the potentially more serious gonococcal aetiology:

1. Treat with a systematic antibiotic: Ceftriaxone 50 mg/kg by intramuscular injection in a single dose (maximum 125 mg); or Kanamycin 25 mg/kg in a single dose (maximum 75 mg).
2. Everyone who cares for the baby must wash their hands thoroughly. The baby's eyes should be washed and tetracycline 1% eye ointment applied to both eyes 6 hourly for 14 days.
3. If no intracellular diplococci are seen in the exudate, or if

discharge persists, there is probably chlamydial infection. Treat with the addition of erythromycin syrup 50 mg/kg/day in four divided doses for 14 days.

Both parents should be examined, investigated and treated.

20
Brucellosis and Melioidosis

BRUCELLOSIS

Brucellosis is a zoonosis, caused by the Gram-negative coccobacilli *Brucella melitensis*, *B. abortus* and *B. suis*, which affects humans if they consume unpasteurized milk or soft cheese from infected cows, goats or camels. It can also be acquired in those working with animals by direct contact or inhalation and is now thought also to have the potential for transfer of human infection through sexual intercourse.

Ingested or inhaled bacilli pass via the blood to multiply within the cells of the reticulo-endothelial system in liver, spleen and bone marrow, where the formation of granulomas is induced.

Clinical brucellosis may take the form of an acute fever with chills or rigors but more often runs a subacute course with sweating, lethargy and splenomegaly; pain and tenderness in the spine result from vertebral osteitis, which is radiologically similar to early spinal tuberculosis. Possible complications include epididymo-orchitis, anicteric hepatitis and endocarditis. Mental depression is common.

The diagnosis is made by blood culture on a special medium, and the plates should be left to incubate for at least 2 and up to 6 weeks before being declared negative. Serological agglutinations tests and CFT are reliable.

The differential diagnosis of brucellosis includes typhoid fever, malaria, Epstein-Barr virus infection, CMV infection, endocarditis of other specific causes, Q fever and miliary tuberculosis.

Brucella organisms are sensitive to tetracyclines, cotrimoxazole, quinolones, rifamcipin and streptomycin. Uncomplicated cases can be given tetracycline 2 g daily (divided) for 21 days or rifampicin 900 mg daily for 30 days (15 mg/kg in children). In endocarditis a combination of streptomycin and rifamcipin has been used successfully.

Brucellosis occurs wherever milk for human consumption is not pasteurized or boiled, and in all pastoral communities.

MELIOIDOSIS

Melioidosis is caused by *Pseudomonas pseudomallei*, a Gram-negative aerobic bacillus which produces a foul smell in culture. It is found especially in surface water and drainage ditches in South-east Asia and Australia, has its reservoir in rodents, and is inhaled or ingested by man.

It can cause:

1. acute septicaemia with sudden death;
2. subacute abscesses in lung (with cavitation similar to tuberculosis), liver or spleen;
3. chronic skin abscesses.

Patients with diabetes mellitus, chronic renal failure, extensive burns and alcoholism are particularly susceptible.

The diagnosis is made by culturing the organism from blood or sputum or by serology (IHA or ELISA IgM).

The differential diagnosis includes malaria, acute thiamine deficiency, tuberculosis, paragonimiasis and systemic fungal infection.

Melioidosis responds to tetracycline, chloramphenicol, ceftazidine or piperacillin.

21
Anthrax, Tularaemia and Plague

ANTHRAX

Anthrax is caused by *Bacillus anthracis*, a Gram-positive aerobe with highly resistant spores. It releases an exotoxin to cause disease and is primarily a zoonosis of domestic animals. The clinical illness varies according to the route of infection.

1. **cutaneous** anthrax results from skin inoculation. A papule becomes a vesicle and then an oedematous pustule covered by a black eschar; regional lymph nodes are enlarged and fever is usual.
2. **gastrointestinal** anthrax results from ingestion of undercooked meat of infected animals and causes septicaemia, abdominal pain and dysentery.
3. **pneumonic** anthrax results from inhalation of spores and causes extensive pneumonitis and mediastinitis of rapid onset with 80–100% mortality.

Diagnosis of anthrax is confirmed by culture of the organisms from skin lesions, blood or sputum. IHA serology is available.

Cutaneous anthrax should be distinguished from a staphylococcal boil, tularaemia, orf and plague, gastrointestinal anthrax from shigellosis, campylobacter jejuni and yersiniosis, and pneumonic anthrax from pneumonic plague, malaria and miliary tuberculosis.

Anthrax responds to crystalline penicillin or tetracycline. Pneumonic cases should receive large doses of parenteral penicillin urgently.

Cutaneous anthrax occurs in many tropical countries and Western Europe; decontamination of animal products, e.g. bone meal, fur, carpets, woollen jackets and drum skins, can be achieved with formaldehyde. Goats, cattle, sheep and yaks are the commonest animal sources. Adequate cooking of meats will prevent gastrointestinal cases.

People at special occupational risk can be vaccinated with Sterne strain and chemoprophylaxis is also possible.

TULARAEMIA

Tularaemia is caused by *Francisella tularensis* a Gram-negative aerobic coccobacillus which causes a zoonosis of rodents and wild game animals. Man may be infected by direct inhalation when catching wild animals or by inoculation by a wide variety of insects – horse and deer flies, fleas, lice, *Aedes* mosquitoes and ticks.

Tularaemia may present as a septicaemic or pneumonic illness or with a painful ulcer at the site of inoculation with regional lymphadenopathy.

The differential diagnosis includes plague, typhus, typhoid, toxoplasmosis, cat-scratch disease and brucellosis. Streptomycin 1 g b.d. for 7 days is the best treatment. Tularaemia occurs in Russia, Mongolia, Japan, Sweden and the North-west USA. A vaccine is used in laboratory personnel and the Russian Army.

PLAGUE

Plague is caused by the Gram-negative aerobic bacillus *Yersinia pseudotuberculosis* var *pestis*. It is a zoonosis primarily of rats transmitted to man by the flea *Xenopsylla cheopis* which can then be passed rapidly from man to man by cases of plague pneumonia.

Flea-borne infection initially causes fever with a grossly enlarged lymph node proximal to the bite, most commonly inguinal; it has an incubation period of 2 to 8 days, and is known as bubonic plague. Septicaemia may then ensue and result in pneumonic plague with extensive pneumonitis and mediastinitis. Meningitis also occurs.

The diagnosis should be suspected from the presence of a painful bubo and confirmed by Gram stain and culture of fluid aspirated from it. Blood culture may also be positive. Polymorph leukocytosis is usual.

Plague can be treated with streptomycin 1 g b.d. i.m. for 10 days or tetracycline; cases of meningitis should receive intravenous chloramphenicol.

Plague as a zoonosis is maintained in rodents, prairie dogs, bobcats and chipmunks and usually transmitted to man from domestic rats. It occurs in East and Central Africa, Madagascar, Bolivia, Brazil, Peru, Vietnam, Myanmar, Mongolia, N. China, Kazakhstan and Southern California.

Community prevention depends on the control of domestic rats, although sudden killing of large numbers encourages their fleas to bite man, so that insecticide must also be used. Individual protection in travellers and those at occupational risk is assisted by the use of Cutter vaccine and possible chemoprophylaxis with doxycycline. Pneumonic cases should be nursed in respiratory isolation by medical and nursing staff who are specifically protected. Bubo fluid and blood is also highly infectious.

22
Rickettsial Diseases

Rickettsial diseases, or rickettsioses, continue to constitute major health problems in many areas of the world in both temperate and tropical regions. They are often difficult to recognize and are generally under-diagnosed and under-reported.

Rickettsial diseases are transmitted by arthropods (ticks, mites, lice and fleas). Direct man-to-man spread does not occur naturally. The main rickettsial diseases, their synonyms and vectors, are shown in Table 22.1.

TYPHUS AND THE SPOTTED FEVER GROUP

Aetiology and epidemiology

Louse-borne typhus
Of the rickettsioses, louse-borne typhus is the only disease that may occur as explosive epidemics in man. The human body louse, *Pediculus humanus humanus*, the vector of the causal *Rickettsia prowazeki*, thrives under socioeconomic conditions where its control is difficult. Recognition and reporting of this disease is, not surprisingly, poor and the worldwide incidence is unknown. Principal foci of disease occur in the highlands of central Africa, including Burundi, Rwanda, Ethiopia and southern Uganda. In South America cases are sporadically reported from the Andean highlands of Bolivia, Equador and Peru. Disease has been reported in the Himalayan region and possibly also in other highland or cold areas of Asia.

The main reservoir of the disease is the convalescent typhus patient who later develops recrudescent Brill-Zinsser disease. *R. prowazeki* infection has been demonstrated in flying squirrels and

Table 22.1 Rickettsial diseases

Disease	Rickettsia sp.	Vector
Spotted fever group		
Rocky mountain spotted fever	R. rickettsia	Tick
Fievre boutonneuse	R. conori	Tick
Kenya tick typhus		
S. African tick fever		
Indian tick typhus		
Queensland tick typhus	R. australis	Tick
North Asian tick typhus	R. sibirica	Tick
Rickettsial pox	R. akari	Mite
Typhus group		
Epidemic typhus	R. prowazeki	Louse
Murine (endemic) typhus	R. mooseri(typhi)	Flea
Shop or urban typhus		
Scrub typhus	R. tsutsugamushi	Mite
Others		
Q. fever	Coxiella burneti	None
Trench fever	Rochalimeae quintana	Louse
Ehrlichiosis	Ehrlichia canis	Tick
	Ehrlichia sennetsu	Tick

other mammals, but these non-human reservoirs probably do not play an important role in the epidemiology of human disease.

Murine typhus
Murine typhus has a wide geographical distribution. Serosurveys have demonstrated high prevalence of seropositivity in areas where the disease is poorly recognized and therefore grossly under-reported.

Murine typhus is a zoonosis, the reservoir of infection being the domestic rat. *R. mooseri (typhi)* is transmitted to man by fleas, principally *Xenopsylla cheopis*, the tropical rat flea. The disease is therefore most common where rats are found in the peri-domestic or work environment where they are attracted to inadequately protected foodstuffs and hence the synonyms 'shop typhus' and 'urban typhus'. *R. mooseri* is not transmitted by the flea bite. Rickettsiae are present in flea faeces which can enter man through a skin abrasion or via the conjunctiva, or by inhalation.

Areas endemic for murine typhus include areas of the southern

USA, the Mediterranean littoral, the Indian subcontinent, the Middle East and South-east Asia.

Scrub typhus
Scrub typhus is a rickettsial disease caused by R. *tsutsugamushi* and transmitted by the bite of larval trombiculid mites. Unlike murine typhus, scrub typhus is a rural disease. Mite infestation occurs in moist, warm terrain consisting of secondary or transitional forms of vegetation that provides good shelter for field rodents on which the larval mites feed. Man is an accidental host when he intrudes into the often sharply localized foci or 'islands' colonized by infected mites.

Scrub typhus occurs throughout much of the Asian-Pacific region. R. *tsutsugamushi* is known to exist in an area extending from northern Japan and the Primorski Krai region in the far north-east of the Asian land mass, to northern Australia in the south, and as far as Afghanistan, Pakistan and neighbouring areas in the west.

Symptomatology in indigenous populations is often non-specific and the prevalence of seropositivity found in sero-surveys of rural populations, e.g. aborigines and Malaysian oil-palm workers, has often demonstrated a previously unrecognized high incidence of scrub typhus in that population.

The infection is maintained by transovarial transmission from one generation of mite to the next. Whilst small mammals may acquire the infection, as each larval mite feeds only once, the mite population, and not the mammalian host, appears to be the reservoir of infection.

Spotted fever
Tick-borne rickettsioses are restricted to foci where major man-biting species of ixodid ticks are suitable vectors and are infected with pathogenic rickettsiae. This most often occurs during occupational or recreational activities in the tick's natural foci. Pets, particularly dogs, may bring ticks into the domestic environment. Cases are usually sporadic, although sharp outbreaks may occur in exposed groups. Infection may be acquired through abrasions in the skin which become contaminated by infected tick faeces or tissue juices. Hence, ticks should not be crushed between the fingers on removal.

The spotted fever group of Rickettsial diseases are widely, though patchily, distributed worldwide. Spotted fever syndromes are often named after the geographical locations in which they were first recognized, e.g. Siberian tick typhus (*R. sibirica*), Queensland tick typhus (*R. australis*). Kenyan tick typhus, South African tick fever and Boutonneuse fever (named after the 'button-like' rash) are all caused by *R. conori*, an illustration of its widespread distribution. Rocky Mountain spotted fever (RMSF), an illness caused by *Rickettsia rickettsi*, although first recognized in this area, is now known to be most commonly found in the eastern states of North America.

An exception to the tick transmission of the spotted fever group occurs with *R. akari* (rickettsialpox), an urban disease which is transmitted to man by the bite of the rodent mite. The reservoir of infection is the domestic mouse.

Clinical features

All the rickettsial diseases have similar clinical features with an underlying pathology of widespread vasculitis, endothelial proliferation, perivascular inflammation, arterial wall necrosis and arteriolar thrombotic occlusion. All organs may be involved by these processes but the brunt of damage is seen in the skin, brain, kidneys and heart.

The severity of disease varies from patient to patient, often unaccountably, although disease tends to be more severe in the elderly. Non-indigenous and therefore non-immune individuals are more likely to develop the recognizable classical clinical disease and it must be stressed that symptomatology in cases in indigenous populations is often very non-specific.

The classical features of rickettsial disease include an incubation period of several days up to two weeks with a sudden onset of general malaise, myalgia, headache, fever and chills, vomiting, together with either diarrhoea or constipation, and photophobia. Deafness may occur, particularly in scrub typhus and RMSF. Generalized lymphadenopathy is common and moderate splenomegaly may be present. In the more severely affected patients, there may be confusion, circulatory collapse and infrequently death associated with haemorrhagic pneumonitis.

Louse-borne typhus

Louse-borne typhus is usually accompanied by a maculopapular rash, which appears one to two days after the onset of the disease. The macules are darkly erythematous, and may be confluent. The rash, often less conspicuous on a dark skin, is most prominent on the trunk and spreads to the limbs but not the face, occasionally becoming haemorrhagic. A petechial or ecchymotic rash may be evident in the most seriously ill, and is often accompanied by digital gangrene.

It is known that in some patients who recover completely from an attack of louse-borne typhus R. prowazeki persists in their tissues and may emerge many years later and cause a recrudescence of the illness, an illness known as Brill-Zinsser disease. The illness tends to be milder and shorter than the original disease. If the patient has moved to a non-endemic area the diagnosis may be missed unless the patient recalls his first attack.

Murine typhus
Murine tuphus is commonly mild and self-limiting and often escapes diagnosis. Murine typhus often occurs without a significant rash but, if present, it is usually sparse, macular and erythematous. The rash does not become haemorrhagic.

Scrub typhus
A skin lesion, known as an eschar, may develop at the site of the infecting mite bite. The eschar, at first a small red papule, develops into a punched-out ulcer, up to 10 mm in diameter, usually covered with a hard black scab. The larval mite vector usually attaches itself to warm, moist areas of the skin, and eschars are often hidden from cursory examination in areas such as the perineum and axillae.

A maculopapular rash is uncommonly seen in patients deriving from the indigenous population. When present, the rash often appears on about the fifth day of fever, appearing first on the trunk and spreading peripherally.

Conjunctival injection is nearly always marked. Lymphadenopathy, at first regional, related to the site of the bite, and later generalized is commonly present. Mental changes, especially confusion and disorientation, although only marked in severe cases are often found. Deafness and tinnitus may occur especially if the illness is left untreated. Bronchitic symptoms are frequent and recent studies in Thailand suggest that scrub typhus may be a common cause of pneumonia.

Spotted fever group
An eschar may develop at the site of the tick bite. In RMSF the rash typically begins as discrete maculopapular lesions and appears on the trunk and extremities on about the fourth day of illness. It may progress to petechial or purpuric lesions and be accompanied by necrosis of the skin, particularly of the digits, nose, ears and scrotum.

Tick typhus gives rise to a maculopapular rash of varying prominence, often starting on the forearm and spreading to the palms, soles and trunk. In severe cases the rash becomes haemorrhagic and gangrene may occur.

In rickettsialpox the initial maculopapular rash becomes vesicular, vesicles forming at the apices of the papules, before the vesicles crust over and desquamate. An eschar may also be present.

Differential diagnosis

A rickettsial disease should be suspected in any febrile patient with a history of potential exposure to a vector, especially if a rash is present.

Differential diagnoses for RMSF include meningococcal septicaemia and haematological causes of purpura. In Africa louse-borne typhus may be confused with relapsing fever. In Southeast Asia scrub typhus must be differentiated from leptospirosis and arboviral infections. Typhoid and malaria may give rise to clinical syndromes similar to rickettsial infections and provide an important differential diagnosis in many areas of the tropics.

Diagnosis

Rickettsiae may be isolated from the patient's blood even during the early stages of the disease. Rickettsiae will grow in embryonated eggs, in tissue culture or in laboratory animals. These techniques are however expensive and often hazardous to laboratory personnel and are not usually practical in routine clinical practice.

Serological techniques relying on the detection of antibodies are usually the mainstay of laboratory diagnosis. Antibodies, however, can usually be detected only late in the illness, and to be useful require a number of serum samples over a period of weeks in order to demonstrate a rise in titre of specific antibody during convalescence.

The Weil-Felix test, where dilutions of sera are titrated against a suspension of *Proteus* bacilli, with agglutination as an end-point, has both low sensitivity and specificity. *Proteus* OXK strain agglutinins are produced in scrub typhus, and OX2 and OX19 agglutinins in other rickettsial diseases. The predictive value of the test increases when acute and convalescent sera can be tested.

More specific serological techniques in use include the complement fixation reaction, using either group or type-specific antigens, microagglutination, indirect agglutination, indirect immunofluorescence and enzyme-linked immunosorbent assays (ELISA). The indirect fluorescent antibody test, although highly sensitive and specific, is impractical for use in rural hospitals not having a fluorescence microscope. A recently developed modification of this test, the indirect immunoperoxidase test, is specific, sensitive, can be easily read with an ordinary light microscope, and provides a permanent slide record of the result. The ELISA is suitable for use either as a fully automated and objective quantitative test in sophisticated laboratories, or a sensitive qualitative, filter paper-based, visual test in field situations.

Techniques which do not require the detection of antibodies are being developed. Amongst these newer techniques are antigen detection, using indirect immunofluorescence, on skin biopsy material and by gas–liquid chromatography of acute sera, techniques which are unlikely to be available outside a sophisticated laboratory.

Treatment

Rickettsiae are very sensitive to both chloramphenicol and to the tetracycline group of drugs. These drugs are rickettsiostatic only, but sufficient immunity develops during treatment to prevent relapse when treatment is withdrawn. Prompt alleviation of symptoms occurs when therapy is given early in the disease. If defervescence has not occurred within 48 hours then the diagnosis must be reviewed. The response will of course be less dramatic if therapy is delayed until severe complications have arisen. Oral therapy only is required unless the patient has intractable vomiting.

Chloramphenicol is usually given as an initial loading dose of 50 mg/kg body weight, this dose being given on subsequent days in divided doses either three or four times daily. Treatment is usually given for one week or until the patient has been afebrile for 24 hours. Chloramphenicol is of course effective against several of the principal differential diagnoses including typhoid and meningococcal disease.

Tetracycline can be given in a similar way to chloramphenicol starting with a loading dose of 25 mg/kg body weight. Doxycycline, a long-acting analogue of oxytetracycline, has been used successfully as a single oral dose of 200 mg in both louse-borne and scrub typhus. Relapses of scrub typhus have occurred when doxycycline is given early in the disease but respond to a further dose.

In critically ill patients first treated late in the course of severe disease there is evidence that high dose steroids, in combination with the appropriate antibiotic, are beneficial.

Prevention and control

Prevention or control of outbreaks of louse-borne typhus in populations such as refugee camps is achieved by vector control. Large populations can be deloused using insecticides such as DDT or malathion.

Murine typhus may be controlled by measures which reduce the rat and flea population, though cultural and economic factors make this impracticable.

Tick and mite-borne typhus cannot be prevented by vector control, except in special, localized circumstances.

Physical methods of personal prophylaxis include application of repellants, such as diethyltoluamide or dimethylphthalate, to clothing and exposed parts of the body and avoidance of areas of known tick or mite infestation.

Vaccines developed in the past are of poor efficacy and are not generally available. Work continues to develop satisfactory vaccines against rickettsial diseases.

Weekly doses of doxycycline 200 mg afford a high degree of protection from scrub typhus. This regimen is often unpleasant to take, may lead to the development of photosensitivity, and has implications for bacterial resistance patterns. This regimen should probably be reserved for special circumstances, such as military operations in highly endemic areas.

COXIELLA BURNETI (Q FEVER)

Aetiology and epidemiology

Coxiella burneti, the aetiological agent of Q fever, is an obligate intracellular (intracytoplasmic) organism belonging to the family *Rickettsiaceae*. Q fever is a zoonosis and organisms may be found in the amniotic fluid, placenta, milk, urine and faeces of infected animals. The organism can survive for long periods as an environmental contaminant and may be found in particular in straw, hides and wool. Persons can become infected without direct contact with animals. Infection is acquired through the inhalation of an infective aerosol or by ingestion of the organism in such sources as unpasteurized milk or contaminated foodstuffs. Transmission occurs rarely via blood transfusion or transplacentally or via the bites of ticks or other arthropods. Person-to-person spread is recorded.

Coxiella burneti has a worldwide distribution with endemic foci most often reported from Australia and parts of Europe.

Clinical features

After entry into the human host there is widespread haematogenous spread of the organism. Infection may be inapparent. Most symptomatic infections are self-limiting, beginning after an incubation period of around 21 days (range 4 to 40+), and lasting 1 to 3 weeks. Fever (38–40 °C, severe headaches, chills and myalgias often begin abruptly. A non-productive cough is present in up to 70% of patients. An evanescent rash is reported in approximately 5% of cases. An acute or more protracted hepatitis occurs in about a third of patients and is associated with mild jaundice, moderate hepatosplenomegaly and right upper quadrant pain abdominal. Mortality in untreated cases is less than 1%.

The infection may be subacute or chronic. *Coxiella burneti* has been recovered from blood more than one year after onset of infection and from placental tissue some 2 to 3 years after initial infection. Chronic infection usually leads to endocarditis particularly in patients with underlying valvular disease. The clinical picture is one of culture-negative endocarditis; however, fever is commonly absent.

Differential diagnosis

The acute illness may resemble that due to legionellosis, mycoplasmic pneumonia, psittacosis and tularaemia. Non-pulmonary infection may suggest brucellosis, typhoid fever, leptospirosis, culture-negative endocarditis, cytomegalovirus and Epstein-Barr virus mononucleosis, and toxoplasmosis.

Diagnosis

The white blood cell count is normal in two thirds of patients. A two- to three-fold increase in transaminase levels occurs in almost all patients.

In cases with pulmonary symptoms the chest radiograph shows patchy areas of consolidation of 'ground glass' appearance in up to 60% of cases. The diagnosis of Q fever pneumonia is usually confirmed serologically. Isolation of the organism requires special techniques and poses a risk to laboratory workers. The microagglutination, complement fixation (CF), and microimmunofluorescence tests as well as the enzyme-linked immunosorbent assay can all be used in making the serological diagnosis. The CF test is most commonly used, a four-fold rise in titre between the acute and convalescent samples being considered diagnostic. In acute Q fever, antibodies to phase II antigens appear; phase I antibodies indicate chronic infection, such as hepatitis or endocarditis. A CF titre of >/= 1 : 200 to phase I antigen is said to be diagnostic of chronic Q fever.

Treatment

The treatment of choice for *Coxiella burneti* pneumonia is tetracycline. Chloramphenicol is also effective. Rifampicin and the quinolones also appear active against *C. burneti*, but experience with them is limited.

HUMAN EHRLICHIOSIS

Ehrlichia canis

Ehrlichia canis is an intraleukocytic organism of the genus *Ehrlichia* and the family *Rickettsiaceae*. Ehrlichiosis has been recognized since 1935 as a tick-borne infection causing acute febrile illness and anaemia in dogs. The importance of canine ehrlichiosis was recognized after the large losses of military dogs working in Vietnam. It is now appreciated that *E. canis* has a worldwide distribution. The first case of human ehrlichiosis was recognized in the United States in 1986 and the first case in Europe has recently been reported from Portugal. It is probably transmitted to man by the bite of an infected tick.

Fever, headache, myalgias, chills, nausea and vomiting have been reported in the majority of patients. A macular rash appears in a third of patients. Arthralgia may be a prominent symptom. Acute renal failure, respiratory failure and encephalitis have all been reported as occurring in human disease.

A majority of patients have leukopenia, thrombocytopenia and abnormal liver function tests. Cerebrospinal fluid pleocytosis and pulmonary infiltrates are common findings.

Diagnosis is based on the demonstration of a four-fold or greater increase in antibody titre to *E. canis*. Intracytoplasmic inclusion bodies may be demonstrated in the white cell series. Tetracycline appears effective in hastening defervescence and recovery.

Ehrlichia sennetsu

This rickettsiosis was initially described in 1954 in a young Japanese man with a mononucleosis-like illness characterized by fever, headache, malaise, conjunctival suffusion, pharyngitis and generalized adenopathy. Hepatosplenomegaly is found in up to 50% of patients.

In addition to Japan, there is serological evidence of the disease in Malaysia and the Philippines. Transmission is probably by arthropod vectors, such as ticks. Treatment with tetracycline is recommended.

Part Four
Diarrhoeal Diseases

23
Diarrhoeal Diseases

A practical approach to the diagnosis and management of diarrhoeal disease in the tropics is to consider three broad symptom categories, namely, acute watery diarrhoea, bloody diarrhoea (dysentery) and chronic diarrhoea.

ACUTE WATERY DIARRHOEA

In developing countries acute watery diarrhoea is the most common manifestation of gastrointestinal disease. Causative organisms include *Vibrio cholera* and *V. parahaemolyticus*, non-typhoid *Salmonellae*, enterotoxigenic and enteropathogenic *Escherichia coli* (ETEC and EPEC), *Clostridium perfringens*, *Cryptosporidium parvum*, along with *Rotavirus*, enteric adenoviruses, and *Norwalk* and related viruses. *Shigella* sp. early in infection may present as acute watery diarrhoea. Diarrhoea may be a presenting feature of many diseases due to non-enteric pathogens, including falciparum malaria.

CHOLERA

Aetiology and epidemiology

Vibrio cholera is a Gram-negative, straight or curved rod with a single polar flagellum. The species is divided into serovars on the basis of its somatic or O antigens. There are more than 60 serovars, but only O:1 causes disease in man. The O:1 serovar is divided into three subtypes: Ogawa, Inaba and Hikojima. Each subtype is divided into two biotypes: classical and El Tor.

V. cholera produces a powerful enterotoxin that causes copious secretory diarrhoea. The enterotoxin produced by *V. cholera* is made up of an A subunit and a B subunit. The B subunit is responsible for binding irreversibly to the host cell surface using the GM1-ganglioside site, facilitated by secretion of neuraminidase which strips neuraminic acid from the host cell's receptor. The A subunit is then internalized by the cell where it stimulates adenylate cyclase resulting in increased secretion of fluid and electrolytes from intestinal cells. In addition to the direct stimulation of adenylate cyclase, cholera toxin may also promote secretion indirectly via release of 5-hydroxytryptamine (5-HT) from enterochromaffin cells. This ability to produce diarrhoea without morphological damage or disruption of absorptive pathways such as sodium-glucose co-transport has been used to therapeutic advantage in oral rehydration therapy (ORT) with glucose-electrolyte solutions.

Infection results from ingestion of organisms in food and water, or directly from person to person by the faecal–oral route. Acute carriers, particularly those with asymptomatic or mild disease, are important in the maintenance and transmission of cholera. The infective dose is high in adults with normal gastric acidity. *Vibrio cholera* can survive in sea water and outbreaks can be related to ingestion of shell fish.

The seventh pandemic of El Tor cholera began in the Celebes Islands in 1961. During the 1960s El Tor cholera began spreading from South-east Asia to Africa, the Middle East and other parts of Asia. In 1991 cholera reached Peru, causing the first outbreak in South America this century. By January 1992, 13 Latin American countries had been affected with over 360 000 cases being reported, accounting for over 70% of all cases reported to WHO in 1991.

Clinical features

The majority of patients with *V. cholera* infection are asymptomatic, or have a mild, self-limiting diarrhoeal illness. The ratio of symptomatic to asymptomatic cases has been estimated to range from 1:7 to 1:100. The proportion of cases that are symptomatic is higher with the classical biotype than with El Tor cholera.

Following an incubation period of 1 to 5 days there is an abrupt onset of copious watery diarrhoea. The diarrhoeal fluid may be white and flecked with mucus, the classic 'rice-water' stool, and fluid loss can lead to rapid and profound dehydration. Fever is unusual, except in children. Vomiting, without associated nausea, may develop, usually after the onset of diarrhoea. Rarely, early ileus leads to shock without diarrhoea (cholera sicca).

Dehydration leads to loss of skin turgor, malaise and obtundation, and the patient is tachycardic, tachypnoeic, hypotensive and often hypothermic. Severe muscle cramps are associated with electrolyte depletion.

With adequate fluid and electrolyte repletion, the disease is self-limiting, and recovery rapid. Important causes of death are hypovolaemic shock, uncompensated metabolic acidosis, and renal failure due to acute tubular necrosis secondary to prolonged hypotension.

Diagnosis

A cholera-like illness may be caused by other organisms, most frequently by enterotoxigenic *E. coli* (ETEC).

Examination of fresh stool under dark-field microscopy may reveal the characteristic motility of the comma-shaped bacilli. Faecal leukocytes and red cells are absent or scanty.

The organism grows well on a variety of media, including MacConkey's agar and thiosulphate-citrate-bile salt-sucrose (TCBS) agar, and can be typed using specific antisera.

Treatment

The prevention and treatment of dehydration and acidosis is the mainstay of the management of cholera. Despite the massive secretory diarrhoea, oral administration of glucose-electrolyte solutions is effective for promoting water and sodium absorption and correcting acidosis. In severe dehydration, when there is profound hypovolaemia and hypotension, intravenous fluid replacement should be used. The type of intravenous fluid is less important than the quantity. Ringer lactate solution or WHO intravenous diarrhoea treatment solution are best matched to the patient's requirement for a slightly hypotonic alkaline fluid with added potassium. Fluid should be infused at a rate of 50 to 100 ml per minute in adults, until a strong radial pulse has been restored. Overhydration of the patient can be avoided by careful clinical observation including monitoring of the central venous pressure, urine output and auscultation of the lung bases.

In children loss of water is relatively greater than loss of electrolytes and complications are more frequent and often more severe. Stupor, coma and convulsions may occur as a result of hypoglycaemia, hypernatraemia or cerebral oedema. Cardiac arrhythmias due to potassium depletion, and pulmonary oedema due to therapeutic overhydration are easily precipitated. Children rehydrated intravenously with Ringer lactate require oral supplementation with potassium and glucose.

Tetracycline in a dose of 50 mg/kg daily, in 6-hourly divided doses, given for 2 days, will reduce the duration and volume of diarrhoea. A single dose of 30 mg/kg of doxycycline is an acceptable alternative. Tetracycline resistant strains have been isolated in Africa and Asia. The quinolone antibiotics appear to be an effective alternative.

Prevention and control

Vaccination campaigns have to date proved disappointing. Vaccination with the current inactivated vaccine gives limited protection. Newer vaccines, including an inactivated oral vaccine (B subunit-killed whole cell vaccine) and a live attenuated strain (CVD 103-HgR) vaccine are undergoing field trials. Cholera vaccination during epidemics can leave the population with a false sense of security and detracts from more important control measures such as the treatment of drinking water. A vaccine will have to confer substantial protection before it becomes a practical public health measure.

Oral tetracycline has been shown to prevent cholera in persons who have been in close contact with the disease. Indiscriminate use of tetracycline will however promote the emergence of resistant strains and has not been shown to affect epidemic spread of disease.

The current South American epidemic of El Tor cholera has been well documented. The overall case-fatality observed has been low (1.06%). This partly reflects the lower virulence of El Tor compared with the classical vibrio but also, without doubt, the remarkable efforts made by all countries exposed to inform their populations and to disseminate the standard treatment procedures to ensure prompt use of rehydration in case management. This low mortality justifies a cholera control strategy based in the short term on health education and early rehydration of patients. Mass chemoprophylaxis has shown itself incapable of containing an epidemic, and has led to the development of multiple antibiotic resistance.

VIBRIO PARAHAEMOLYTICUS

Vibrio parahaemolyticus causes acute diarrhoea and is usually associated with consumption of contaminated raw fish or shellfish. The illness is generally mild and short-lived. The organism is sensitive to several antibiotics, including tetracycline, but there is no evidence that antimicrobial therapy has a place in the management of this infection.

NON-TYPHOIDAL SALMONELLOSIS

Aetiology and epidemiology

Salmonellae continue to be one of the main causes of food-borne illness worldwide. *Salmonellae* are Gram-negative, motile, rod-shaped bacteria. They are ubiquitous among domestic and wild warm-blooded animals and almost all serovars cause illness in man. Salmonellosis in man is usually due to the consumption of contaminated food. The infective dose is high and salmonellae need to multiply in food to be present in sufficient numbers to cause infection. Secondary spread may occur directly via the faecal–oral route. Water-borne infection is rare. A chronic carrier state in man can occur, and may be associated with gall-bladder disease. Adult schistosomes harbour salmonellae and chronic schistosomiasis can therefore lead to a chronic carrier state.

Invasion of the lamina propria is essential for the production of diarrhoea. Enterotoxins, not dissimilar to those produced by *V. cholera*, are produced. The adenyl cyclase system may also be activated by prostaglandins produced by polymorphonuclear leukocytes.

Clinical features

Asymptomatic infection is common. After an incubation period of 12 to 72 hours most symptomatic cases have an onset with fever and chills. Diarrhoea and, less commonly, vomiting develops, and is often accompanied by abdominal cramps, fever and general malaise. Diarrhoea is loose or watery, often containing mucus, and is occasionally blood-stained. Bloody diarrhoea indicates colonic involvement. Most illnesses follow a mild to moderate self-limiting course with resolution of symptoms within 3 to 5 days, but on occasion septicaemia will develop.

Patients with chronic schistosomiasis are particularly prone to salmonella septicaemia. Individuals with sickle-cell anaemia may develop a salmonella osteomyelitis. Symptoms arising from focal suppurative complications (e.g. in bone, joints, spleen, cardiac valve, aorta) may be subacute and develop weeks or months after primary infection. Infections with salmonellae, especially *Salmonella typhimurium*, occur more often in HIV-positive individuals than in the seronegative population and are more likely to be bacteraemic.

Diagnosis

Confirmation of the diagnosis depends on isolation of the salmonella from faeces, blood or other material.

Treatment

Although antibiotics have been used to treat non-typhoidal salmonella gastroenteritis, there is debate as to whether they convincingly alter the rate of clinical recovery. Antibiotic therapy has been demonstrated to increase the incidence and duration of intestinal carriage by suppressing the normal bowel flora.

Patients with underlying debility or immunosuppression and cases with septicaemia do however benefit from antibiotic treatment. Multiple drug resistance is increasingly common and, whenever possible, treatment should be guided by *in vitro* sensitivities. Treatment with chloramphenicol can be given 50 mg/kg daily, in four divided doses, for up to 14 days. Ampicillin or amoxycillin can be used in a dose of 50–100 mg/kg daily in divided doses, orally or parenterally, for 10 to 14 days. Where available, ciprofloxacin, up to 750 mg orally twice daily for 7 to 28 days, is considered the drug of choice.

Relapse after treatment is common in HIV-infected patients, whose infections are often bacteraemic, and chronic suppressive therapy may be required to control infection.

ENTEROTOXIGENIC *ESCHERICHIA COLI* (ETEC)

Aetiology and epidemiology

ETEC has a worldwide distribution and is an important cause of gastroenteritis in infants and traveller's diarrhoea in adults. ETEC is non-invasive and produces both a heat-labile and heat-stable toxins. The heat-labile toxin is almost identical to cholera enterotoxin.

A relatively large inoculum is required to produce disease. Faecal contamination of food, and to lesser extent water, is the usual source of ETEC. Direct person-to-person transmission of ETEC is uncommon.

Clinical features

Following an incubation period of 1 to 3 days, which is dependent on the size of the infecting dose, ETEC infection produces a self-limiting illness of diarrhoea and cramping abdominal pain lasting 4 to 7 days. In children dehydration and acidosis will supervene if water and electrolyte losses are not promptly replaced. Fever is uncommon and other than dehydration there are no serious complications.

Diagnosis

Diagnosis requires specialized laboratory facilities to detect enterotoxins in culture filtrates. The ability of ETEC to produce enterotoxin depends on the possession of a bacterial plasmid. DNA probes are now available to detect these plasmids in faeces without any necessity to first culture the organisms.

Treatment

Oral rehydration with glucose-electrolyte solution is effective. The treatment and prevention of traveller's diarrhoea caused by ETEC is discussed in Chapter 35.

ENTEROPATHOGENIC *ESCHERICHIA COLI* (EPEC)

The pathogenesis of diarrhoea due to EPEC is unknown. They are not invasive, nor do they produce any currently identifiable toxin.

In the tropics diarrhoeal disease caused by EPEC is most common between the ages of 6 and 18 months, the time of weaning. After a short incubation period there is abrupt onset of watery diarrhoea, usually associated with vomiting and fever. Treatment is supportive, with careful attention to fluid and electrolyte replacement.

CLOSTRIDIUM PERFRINGENS

Aetiology and epidemiology

Clostridium perfringens infection has a worldwide distribution. Type A strains produce a heat-labile enterotoxin. Soil or faecal contamination of food with *C. perfringens* leads to the production of enterotoxin associated with the sporulation of the organism.

Clostridium perfringens Type C has been associated with cases of necrotizing enterocolitis. This type produces large amounts of beta-toxin which has a lethal and necrotizing effect on tissues. It is prevalent in Papua New Guinea where it gives rise to a condition called 'pig bel'.

Clinical features

Symptoms of food-borne infection due to Type A strain usually occur 8 to 24 hours after ingestion of heavily contaminated food. The usual symptoms are diarrhoea and severe abdominal pain, whereas fever and vomiting are unusual. The occasional reports of sporadic illness, in which symptoms developed within 2 hours, point to a role of preformed toxin.

Type C strains of *C. perfringens* can give rise to an acute infection varying in severity from a short-lived attack of diarrhoea to a rapidly fatal necrotizing enteritis. The enterotoxin is inactivated by proteolytic enzymes in the intestine. Susceptible people are those in whom production of these enzymes is low because of their nutritional status or whose enzymes are impaired by inhibitors in the diet. In Papua New Guinea sweet potato, a local dietary staple, contains an inhibitor of trypsin. The disease is characterized by the sudden development of severe abdominal pain, bloody diarrhoea, vomiting and shock. Segmental full-thickness necrosis of the bowel occurs, the brunt of disease falling on the ileum.

Diagnosis

The organism can be demonstrated in the stool and small bowel contents.

Treatment

Treatment of Type A disease is supportive. Necrotizing enteritis requires treatment with nasogastric intubation and aspiration and with intravenous fluid and electrolyte replacement. Antibiotics including chloramphenicol and ampicillin, and administration of Type C antitoxins, are beneficial. Surgical intervention is required for persistent toxicity or when there is evidence of intestinal obstruction. In these circumstances mortality is high. In recovered patients chronic partial obstruction may develop as healing leads to scarring and intestinal malabsorption may ensue.

Prevention and control

Health education and food hygiene measures are paramount. *Clostridium perfringens* Type C toxoid vaccine, two doses 3 to 4 months apart, has been shown to prevent the disease.

DYSENTERY

The appearance of blood in the stools suggests an invasive process in the colon. The major organisms responsible for dysentery include *Shigella* sp., enteroinvasive *E. coli* (EIEC), enterohaemorrhagic *E. coli* (EHEC), *Entamoeba histolytica*, *Schistosoma* sp. and *Trichuris trichuria*. *Salmonella* sp., *Campylobacter jejuni* and *Yersinia enterocolitica* may give rise to blood-stained stools.

SHIGELLOSIS

Aetiology and epidemiology

The four species of the genus *Shigella* (*dysenteriae*, *flexneri*, *boydii* and *sonnei*) cause a wide spectrum of illness from watery diarrhoea to fulminant dysentery. The most severe disease is caused by *S. dysenteriae* Type 1. *S. flexneri* strains are somewhat less virulent, whereas *S. boydii* and *S. sonnei* usually cause a self-limiting febrile, watery diarrhoeal illness. The manifestations of dysentery are due to an inflammatory colitis secondary to bacterial invasion of the colonic epithelial cells and, in *S. dysenteriae* Type 1, cytotoxin production leading to epithelial cell death.

Shigellosis has a worldwide distribution, but *S. dysenteriae* Type 1 and *S. flexneri* predominate in developing countries, in association with poverty, overcrowding, poor levels of personal hygiene, inadequate water supplies and malnutrition. Over the past two decades major epidemics of *S. dysenteriae* Type 1 infection have been documented in Latin America, Central Africa (Zaire,

Rwanda, Central African Republic), Asia (Burma, Vietnam, Thailand) and the Indian sub-continent (India, Bangladesh).

In developing countries shigellosis is a paediatric disease; the majority of patients are less than 10 years of age, and most are younger than 5 years. Prospective studies in developing countries have observed incidence rates of 750 to 2000/1000 children per year. During disease epidemics as many as one in ten people will become infected, and as many as 10 to 15% of these will die.

Humans are the only important reservoir of infection. The major mode of transmission is person to person, facilitated by the need for a very small inoculum to give rise to disease. Seasonal patterns of transmission are observed. In Bangladesh the infection peaks in the hot dry season. In south India peak incidence is in the monsoon season, whereas in Guatemala the peak is just before and during the early part of the rainy season.

Clinical features

The initial manifestations of shigellosis are fever and malaise. Watery diarrhoea develops, and in some patients it progresses to bloody diarrhoea or dysentery within hours or days, in part depending on the infecting species. The classical dysenteric stool is a small amount of blood and mucus, but patients commonly pass formed stool mixed with blood and mucus. Stool frequency is usually 10 to 25 per day. Vomiting is common and the patient is prostrated. Abdominal cramps can be severe and tenesmus due to proctitis can lead to rectal prolapse, especially in the very young. Anorexia is a general finding in shigellosis and there is a significant decrease in food intake which persists into the convalescent period. This, in addition to protein loss through diarrhoea, can lead to a marked negative nitrogen balance resulting in the progression of marginal malnutrition to overt protein-energy malnutrition.

Toxic megacolon and perforation can develop in severe infections, leading to peritonitis and septicaemia. Haemolytic-uraemic syndrome can develop in children, often towards the end of the first week of symptomatic infection, as bowel symptoms are beginning to improve. Large volume fluid loss is not a problem, but hyponatraemia may develop secondary to inappropriate antidiuretic hormone secretion.

Diagnosis

Stool microscopy demonstrates numerous pus cells but few bacilli. Definitive diagnosis depends on recovery of the organism from stool, which is facilitated when more than one selective culture medium is employed.

Treatment

Volume losses are not great in shigellosis and fluid replacement can be provided by ORT. Disease of mild or moderate severity is usually self-limiting and requires no other specific treatment. Because of the severe complications that can follow *S. dysenteriae* Type 1 infection, antibiotics are usually given. There is widespread resistance to drugs such as ampicillin and co-trimoxazole, and resistant strains have been treated with nalidixic acid, or more recently the 4-fluoroquinolone drugs. Resistance to nalidixic acid has already been encountered, and potential adverse effects on cartilage are a relative contraindication for using quinolone antibiotics in children.

Prevention and control

The most effective way to reduce the incidence of shigellosis is to ensure proper washing of hands following defaecation, and adequate disposal of faeces. The prevention of shigellosis is closely linked to efforts to improve the economic and social conditions of people living in areas where shigellosis is now endemic.

ENTEROHAEMORRHAGIC *ESCHERICHIA COLI* (EHEC)

EHEC releases potent cytotoxins or verotoxins bearing a close resemblance to Shiga toxin of *S. dysenteriae* Type 1.

These infections are now recognized to be an important problem in North America, Europe and the cone of South America. Their relative importance in the rest of the world is not yet established.

The spectrum of disease caused by EHEC is wide and includes asymptomatic infection, mild non-bloody diarrhoea, and a dysentery-like illness. There is a strong association with the development of haemolytic-uraemic syndrome (HUS) in children. A large proportion of children who develop HUS first present with diarrhoea, which is often bloody, and may precede the onset of HUS by up to 3 weeks. Treatment with antibiotics does not prevent progress to HUS, and the use of antimotility agents appears to increase the risk of HUS developing.

ENTEROINVASIVE *ESCHERICHIA COLI* (EIEC)

EIEC penetrate gut mucosa and multiply within epithelial cells of the colon, causing a dysenteric illness. These organisms are of worldwide distribution, and they tend to affect older children and adults rather than infants.

CAMPYLOBACTER ENTERITIS

Aetiology and epidemiology

Campylobacter jejuni, a motile, comma-shaped, micro-aerophilic, Gram-negative rod, is the species recognized as being a major human pathogen in both western and developing countries. In developing countries, where children are repeatedly exposed, carrier rates reach 40% in asymptomatic children, and disease occurs primarily in the very young.

The infective dose is small, and infection may be by person-to-person spread or from contaminated food or water. Both tissue invasion and cytolytic exotoxin contribute to pathological changes, primarily affecting the small bowel but commonly extending to the colon.

Clinical features

There is an average incubation period of 2 to 4 days. Symptomatic disease may range from a mild diarrhoeal illness through to fulminant dysentery. Fever, headache and myalgias may precede the diarrhoea. Localized abdominal pain may mimic acute appendicitis. Tenesmus is common in patients with large bowel inflammation and bloody stools. Vomiting is not a conspicuous feature of the illness, but almost all patients experience nausea. Severe diarrhoea seldom lasts for more than a few days, but loose stools, abdominal pain and malaise may be more prolonged. A brief relapse is not uncommon.

Complications include metastatic infection (e.g. meningitis, endocarditis), gastrointestinal haemorrhage, pancreatitis and toxic megacolon. Reactive arthritis, erythema nodosum, haemolytic-uraemic syndrome, and Guillain-Barré syndrome have all been reported following *Campylobacter* infection. In HIV-infected persons infection may involve the biliary tree.

Diagnosis

Campylobacter can be isolated from stool on selective media with conditions for micro-aerobic culture. With dark-field or phase-contrast microscopy the skilled observer may observe the organisms by virtue of their characteristic morphology and motility. If organisms are plentiful they may be recognized in a Gram-stained faecal preparation.

Treatment

Supportive treatment with fluid and electrolyte replacement is the mainstay of treatment. When a patient is acutely ill at the time of bacteriological diagnosis it is appropriate to give a short course of antibiotic. Erythromycin is the drug of first choice and an adult dose of 500 mg three times daily for 5 days is appropriate. Ciprofloxacin is an alternative treatment, although resistance to both erythromycin and ciprofloxacin has been observed, particularly in Thailand.

YERSINIA ENTEROCOLITICA

Yersinia enterocolitica, an anaerobic, Gram-negative coccoid bacillus, is rapidly emerging worldwide as a significant enteric pathogen, but is found most frequently in cooler climates. The disease is a zoonosis, and is acquired by man via food and water contaminated with infected animal faeces. *Y. enterocolitica* gives rise to ileal and caecal inflammation and an illness characterized by fever, abdominal pain and diarrhoea which may be watery and bloodstained. Post-infection manifestations include erythema nodosum and reactive arthritis. Antibiotic treatment is not required for uncomplicated enterocolitis.

CHRONIC DIARRHOEA

The well-defined causes of chronic diarrhoea are infection with enteropathogenic *E. coli* (EPEC), *Giardia*, *Cryptosporidium*, *Strongy*-

loides stercoralis and tropical sprue. A specific cause of chronic diarrhoea in children in the tropics is often not identified, and it is likely that a variety of factors act together to give rise to chronic childhood diarrhoea, e.g, parasitic infection, altered microflora of the small intestine, impaired immune and non-immune barrier functions in the small intestine secondary to undernutition, etc.

Post-infective tropical malabsorption (tropical sprue)

Aetiology and epidemiology
Tropical sprue has been documented in South-east Asia, particularly India and Nepal, in the Caribbean, parts of Central and northern South America and Queensland. Although described in Africa, its occurrence is rare in this continent.

Tropical sprue is a syndrome of malabsorption occurring among residents of or visitors to these areas of the tropics and subtropics. Its epidemiological pattern suggests that exposure to an infectious or other environmental agent or agents is crucial. Persistent colonization of the proximal portion of the small intestine with coliform bacteria has been demonstrated in many, but not all, patients with sprue. It has been suggested that patients who develop sprue may have a primary defect in the ability to regenerate crypt cells.

Histopathological examination of the mucosa of the small intestine shows a wide variety of changes, none of which are specific. Changes include a variable degree of villous shortening and crypt hyperplasia, infiltration of the lamina propria with inflammatory cells, especially lymphocytes and plasma cells, and prominent infiltration of the damaged absorptive epithelium with lymphocytes.

Clinical features
The most usual form of sprue has an acute onset, runs a short self-limiting course, and remits on leaving an endemic area. Another, now less common form, is seen particularly in India, and was once common in overland travels to India and the East. This has a slow insidious onset, runs a chronic progressive course, and gives rise to chronic malabsorption and emaciation.

Features of the acute form include acute onset diarrhoea, abdominal colic and distension, progressing to steatorrhoea with the malabsorption of fat, xylose and vitamin B_{12}. In the chronic form the onset of steatorrhoea is more insidious, and is associated with the development of glossitis and stomatitis, nausea, anaemia, peripheral oedema, osteoporosis and asthenia with marked weight loss and emaciation. The anaemia is associated with deficiencies of iron, folic acid and vitamin B_{12}. It is normoblastic in the early stages, but is frankly megaloblastic in established disease.

Diagnosis
None of the cardinal features of sprue are specific, and the diagnosis is clinical, based on travel history and exclusion of other causes of malabsorption.

Treatment
The object of treatment is to eradicate any chronic bacterial colonization of the bowel and to restore any deficiencies caused by malabsorption.

A broad spectrum antibiotic such as tetracycline is give 1 g twice daily for at least 10 to 14 days, although prolonged treatment is required for some individuals. It is also conventional to give folic acid and vitamin B_{12}.

Response to treatment is often rapid. In patients with the more chronic form treatment may need to be continued for some months before marked improvement is seen.

Note. For a discussion of viral gastroenteritis, see Blacklow *et al.* (1991).

Part Five
Viral Diseases

24
Arboviruses

Arbovirus (arthropod-borne virus) infections comprise a number of taxonomic and antigenic groupings of diseases which are mostly primarily zoonoses. Classification is complicated by the facts that:

1. not all are, in fact, arthropod-borne;
2. neither the taxonomic group nor the antigenic structure necessarily predicts the usual clinical syndrome in man;
3. the same virus in different countries and different individuals may produce a different clinical picture;
4. the names of the viruses reflect the original place of discovery and not the current geographical area of risk.

There are three principal clinical syndromes:

1. fever with rash, often with joint and muscle pain;
2. haemorrhagic fever;
3. encephalitis.

The common examples of these syndromes are shown in Table 24.1.

The majority of these viruses have mosquitoes as the vector insect; many have domestic or wild animals as 'amplifying' hosts in which a multiplying viraemia causes no serious disease in the young animal but creates a pool of infection for vector transmission, through which man becomes an incidental host.

Yellow fever is caused by a flavivirus which is maintained in nature in jungle monkeys by mosquito vectors (*Stegomyia, Haemagogus*) in which transovarial transmission of the virus also occurs. Human encroachment into rain forest where the infection exists results in sporadic cases of illness, but epidemic human disease occurs only when *Aedes* mosquitoes (e.g. *Ae. aegypti*) with an

Table 24.1 Clinical syndromes caused by arboviruses

Fever	Haemorrhagic fever	Encephalitis
Dengue	Yellow	Japanese
West Nile	Haemorrhagic dengue	Western equine
Sandfly	Lassa	Eastern equine
Rift Valley	Congo Crimea	St Louis
Oropouche	Rift Valley	California
Chikungunya		La Crosse
O'nyong'nyong		Murray Valley
Ross River		Kyasanur
		European tick-borne
		Siberian tick-borne
		Colorado tick-borne
		'Louping ill'

urban breeding cycle transmit the virus from man to man. Potential for this exists in sub-Saharan Africa and northern South America, with recent epidemic spread especially having occurred in Cameroon and Nigeria.

After an incubation period of 3 to 6 days, many patients suffer only a mild febrile illness for 2 to 3 days from which they recover. Some develop a more severe syndrome with muscle pain, headache and albuminuria; again some patients recover spontaneously. In the most severe cases, perhaps after respite from fever for a day or two, high fever returns with nausea, vomiting, severe head and muscle pain, a flushed face, albuminuria, oliguria, jaundice and a bleeding diathesis, with myocarditis. In such cases there is leukopenia, severe disturbance of blood clotting, markedly raised liver cell enzymes and serum bilirubin, hypoglycaemia and uraemia. The differential diagnosis includes severe viral hepatitis, *P. falciparum* malaria, relapsing fever, leptospirosis and other viral haemorrhagic fevers. Diagnosis can be made by viral isolation from blood or a serum ELISA test.

No specific treatment exists for yellow fever; severe cases require intensive supportive management. The mortality in epidemic diseases is from 20 to 50%, since such treatment is rarely available.

Yellow fever is fully preventable by vaccination; live attenuated 17 D strain virus provides immunity for life after a single injection, but WHO regulations require boosting injections every 10 years for certification. This vaccine should not be given to pregnant women or immuno-compromised subjects. In endemic countries the vaccine is currently employed in response to the crisis of an epidemic; in future routine vaccination of all children should be attempted. Measures to control urban breeding of *Aedes* mosquitoes also contribute to control of the infection. Travel between infected areas is controlled by WHO regulations.

Dengue fever is caused by a flavivirus of which four principal serological strains exist. It is maintained in nature in primates by various species of *Aedes* mosquito and transmitted to man by urban *Aedes aegypti*. It has a wide distribution in the Caribbean, Central and northern South America, East and West-Africa, India, South-east Asia and the Pacific Islands.

After an incubation period of about 4 days, a viraemic illness lasting 4 to 7 days occurs. In small children this may present as upper respiratory tract infection; in non-immune older children and adults, there is a sudden onset of high fever with headache, painful eye movement, muscle and joint pain, red eyes and a puffy face, nausea and vomiting, general lymphadenopathy and a fine pale maculo-papular or morbilliform rash. Splenomegaly is unusual. A few patients suffer a second milder illness for 1–2 days after an interval of 2–3 days, and some develop post-viral depression or chronic fatigue symptoms. Treatment of uncomplicated dengue fever is symptomatic, with oral fluids and analgesics.

Dengue haemorrhagic fever occurs in tropical America, the Caribbean and South-east Asia in infants of immune mothers and in children over 1 year in second and subsequent infections, especially if the virus strain is new to the individual. Sensitized monocytes, in which the virus multiplies, induce release of cytokines (e.g. tumour necrosis factor (TNF)) which cause increased vascular permeability, focal haemorrhage and major extravasation of circulating fluid, leading to shock. A child with this form of dengue is restless and shocked, may have haemorrhagic pleural effusions, a bleeding diathesis, and thrombocytopenia, with a markedly raised haematocrit. Intensive intravenous supportive treatment with Ringer's solution, dextran, plasma or whole blood is required, together with oxygen and sedation (e.g. with chloral hydrate).

Prevention of dengue depends on the reduction of indoor and peridomestic *Aedes* breeding by insecticide spraying and health education. Sleeping nets are not of great value since the vector bites by day; vaccine development has been hampered by the unusual immunological relationship of complicated haemorrhagic illness to previous exposure to other virus strains.

Most of the other uncomplicated arbovirus fevers are clinically very similar to non-haemorrhagic dengue fever. **West Nile fever** is transmitted by *Culex* mosquitoes and has a reservoir in many mammals and birds. It occurs widely in Africa, Asia, southern Europe and Russia. **Sandfly fever** is transmitted by Phlebotomine sandflies and occurs in North Africa, Arabia, southern Europe and Central Asia. **Oropouche fever** in Brazil and Trinidad is transmitted by *Culicoides* midges. **Chikungunya** has a primate reservoir in sub-Saharan Africa, India and South-east Asia and is transmitted by *Aedes* mosquitoes. Joint pain is a special feature. **O'nyong'nyong** occurs in Uganda and is transmitted by anophelines. **Ross River fever** occurs in Australia, Papua New Guinea and the Pacific Islands, and is transmitted from wild vertebrates by *Aedes* and *Culex* mosquitoes. Joint pain is common with this virus, and arthritis may persist for some weeks.

Arboviruses which commonly cause encephalitis are shown in Table 24.2; in all over 20 viruses of this category are known to have the potential to cause encephalitis. They are zoonoses especially of young animals, which are asymptomatic but viraemic and so transmit the viruses to the vector insect. Infected humans are also viraemic prior to the onset of the prodromal illness, which lasts for 2–3 days and consists of banal headache, fever and malaise. Of those infected 95 to 99% recover without complications. A small minority, especially young non-immune children and elderly people whose immunity has declined, develop encephalitis, with increasing headache, delirium, clouding of consciousness, hyperreflexia, focal muscle weakness and often, in children, repeated major convulsions. The mortality of established encephalitis varies from under 10% with St Louis virus to over 25% in Japanese encephalitis and up to 50% with the relatively rare Eastern American virus. Autopsies of fatal cases show marked perivascular monocyte and lymphocyte infiltration in the brain, and large numbers of viruses in neuronal cells both in brain and spinal cord. CSF examination in life shows increases in lymphocytes and protein and pressure may be raised. Up to 50% of survivors of severe encephalitis have neurological sequelae – dystonia, ataxia, spasticity and mental impairment.

Definitive diagnosis is made by the demonstration of IgM antibodies in serum and CSF by ELISA. If possible, herpes virus

Table 24.2 Arboviral encephalitis

	Name	Vector	Animal host	Geography
F	Japanese	*Culex*	Water birds Pigs Bovines	S.E. Asia Japan India Nepal Sri Lanka
T	Eastern	*Aedes*	Birds	E. USA Gulf of Mexico S. America
T	Western	*Culex*	Birds	W. USA and Canada
T	Venezuelan	Various mosquitoes	Horses Small mammals	S. and C. America Florida SW USA
F	St Louis	*Culex*	Birds	USA
F	Murray Valley	*Culex*	Birds	Australia PNG
F	Siberian tick	*Ixodes*	Small mammals	E. Siberia
F	European tick	*Ixodes*	Small mammals	E. and S. Central Europe
F	Kyasanur tick	*Haemophysalis*	Small mammals	India (Local)
F	'Louping ill'	*Ixodes*	Small mammals and sheep	UK
B	California	*Aedes*	Small mammals	W. USA
B	La Crosse	*Aedes*	Small mammals	Mid W. USA Mid E. USA

F = flavivirus
T = togavirus
B = bunyavirus

encephalitis should be excluded, since it is amenable to specific treatment, whereas arbovirus encephalitis is not. Supportive treatment includes antipyretics, anticonvulsants and care of the airway. Differential diagnoses to be considered in tropical countries include rabies, cerebral cysticercosis, bacterial meningitis and falciparum malaria.

Prevention and control of arbovirus encephalitis requires:

1. use of vaccines where available (e.g. Japanese virus);
2. control of peridomestic mosquito breeding;
3. manipulation of breeding seasons of domestic amplifying host animals to avoid seasonal increases in vector insect population (e.g. pigs).

Japanese encephalitis, the commonest of these illnesses, occurs in seasonal epidemics, especially in children, towards the end of monsoon seasons in India (especially Bihar and West Bengal), the Nepal terai, Bangladesh, Myanmar, Vietnam, Thailand, West and East Malaysia, Indonesia, southern Japan, and southern China (including occasional cases in Hong Kong). The vector is most often dusk-feeding *Culex tritaeniorhynchus* and amplifying hosts include herons, egrets, piglets, water buffalo calves and young horses. There are several effective vaccines, e.g. inactivated virus in mouse-brain, live attenuated virus in hamster kidney cells, but their expense prevents large scale use in the populations at risk.

In the United States, the commonest infection is due to **St Louis virus**, with passerine birds (e.g house sparrows) as the amplifying hosts, and various *Culex* mosquitoes as vectors. It occurs in summer outbreaks in the southern states, and has a mortality of 7% in symptomatic cases, mainly in elderly subjects.

In Australia, **Murray Valley virus** causes encephalitis in children in the summer months in the Murray and Darling valleys, with water birds being the amplifying hosts and *Culex* the vector. The same virus occurs in Papua New Guinea.

Tick-borne encephalitis is caused by at least four viruses; that found in South-east Europe can be prevented by a good inactivated vaccine and avoidance of the forest habitat in summer.

Viral haemorrhagic fevers (VHFs) are exemplified by yellow fever (see above); other important viruses are shown in Table 24.3.

Lassa fever occurs in Nigeria and other countries in West Africa. The virus is excreted in the urine of the rodent *Mastomys natalensis* and transmitted directly by aerosol to man. After an incubation period of 7 to 18 days, the illness varies in severity from a mild 'influenza-like' syndrome through diarrhoea to a severe prostrating illness with high fever, exudative pharyngitis, conjunctivitis, bleeding from gums and nose and into skin, potentially complicated by haemorrhagic pleural effusions, myopericarditis, encephalitis, abortion in pregnant women and respiratory distress syndrome.

Laboratory investigations show a raised haematocrit, raised liver cell enzymes and reduced platelet count; specific diagnosis is made by ELISA or IFAT demonstration of IgM antibodies. Intensive supportive treatment may be needed and, if possible, specific antiviral treatment with high doses of intravenous ribavirin should be given. Control of Lassa virus in the field is

Table 24.3 Viral haemorrhagic fevers

Name	Geography	Tranmission to man
Argentine	Argentina (humid pampas)	Rodent urine
Bolivian	Bolivia (plains)	Rodent urine
Lassa	W. Africa	Rodent urine Nosocomial
Ebola	E. and C. Africa	? (Nosocomial)
Hantaan (HFRS)	E. Asia Europe	Vole and field mouse urine
Congo–Crimea (CCHF)	C. and S. Africa Arabia E. Europe Russia Georgia Ukraine	From sheep, goats and man via *Ixodes* ticks (also nosocomial);
Rift Valley (RVF)	Africa (Mauritania Madagascar Egypt)	From ruminants, esp. camels by aerosol; perhaps via mosquitoes, fleas and ticks

problematical; the risks of nosocomial infection have been exaggerated and attach only to the patient's blood, and not to droplet or aerosol spread.

The virus of **Congo–Crimea haemorrhagic fever** (CCHF) has a wide distribution in Russia, the Balkans, Arabia, and extensively in Africa. It is transmitted from sheep and goats to man by Ixodid ticks; in the 1990 Haj at Mecca this occurred when large numbers of sheep and goats were slaughtered for food. Severe cases are clinically similar to yellow fever; ribavirin treatment may be effective.

Rift Valley fever (RVF) has occurred in epidemic form in Egypt but has also spread as far as Mauritania and Madagascar. The method of dissemination from sick ruminant animals, notably camels on trading routes, is uncertain and may be by direct aerosol or through various insect vectors. A severe haemorrhagic fever, without jaundice, may occur. Ribavirin treatment is beneficial.

Ebola virus in Zaire and southern Sudan is clinically similar to Lassa fever. The mode of transmission is unknown and ribavirin treatment is not effective.

Hantaan virus causes 'haemorrhagic fever with renal syndrome' (HFRS); it is disseminated in rodent urine and has been found in Korea, Japan, China and Europe. Acute renal failure results from hypovolaemia due to extravasation of fluid; conservative renal management often results in diuresis and recovery. The response of this virus to ribavirin is good.

25
Acquired Immunodeficiency Syndrome

Acquired Immunodeficiency Syndrome (AIDS) is a disease caused by Human Immunodeficiency Virus (HIV) and was first recognized in 1981. The disease has spread to all continents and represents a major challenge to health workers around the world.

First reported in the USA in 1981, AIDS was reported from Africa in 1982. AIDS remains under-reported as surveillance for the syndrome is poorly developed and because diagnostic capabilities for AIDS and associated opportunistic diseases are often limited. The World Health Organization clinical case definition for AIDS was intended mainly as an epidemiological tool for hospital surveillance of AIDS cases, but in practice has proved less than 60% sensitive. Clinical definitions which optimize sensitivity and specificity for AIDS are being developed for both diagnostic and epidemiological purposes. Worldwide, an estimated 8 to 10 million persons were infected with the HIV virus by mid-1990 and 263 000 AIDS cases had been reported from 156 countries.

The main modes of transmission in America and Europe are penetrative sexual contact in homosexuals and bisexuals, and the sharing of virus contaminated needles among intravenous drug abusers, although there is increasing concern of heterosexual spread. Homosexuality and intravenous drug abuse are rarely acknowledged by Africans and it would appear that in Africa spread has been by heterosexual sex and by congenital or perinatal transmission from mother to child. It has been suggested that heterosexual spread in Africa has been more rapid than amongst heterosexuals in the developed world partly because of increased frequency of different sexual partners. Evidence is growing that genital ulcerations, and perhaps other sexually transmitted diseases as well, increase the risk of sexual transmission of HIV infection.

Infection with the HIV virus is often initially asymptomatic. A seroconversion syndrome mimicking an infectious mononucleosis-like syndrome may appear soon after viral infection. Generalized lymphadenopathy may persist for months in patients who are otherwise asymptomatic. After an incubation period of months to years, HIV-infected persons develop opportunist infections as evidence of deteriorating immune competence. This stage may last several years but progresses inexorably to overwhelming infections or neoplasms which lead to death.

CLINICAL FEATURES

Cutaneous manifestations

Recurrent bacterial, viral and fungal infections of the skin occur with increased frequency in AIDS. Examples of cutaneous manifestations are listed below:

> Multidermatomal and necrotic herpes zoster, severe genital herpes and extensive molluscum contagiosum are common manifestations.
> Seborrhoeic dermatitis, refractory to treatment, extensive tinea corporis and worsening psoriasis are also features.
> Cutaneous candidiasis, involving the genitocrural fold, perianal region, axillae and hands and feet.
> 'Pruritic maculo-papular eruption'.
> Cutaneous lesions of pellagra in patients with chronic AIDS-related diarrhoea.
> Cutaneous manifestations of Kaposi's sarcoma.

AIDS-associated intestinal infections

Oral and oesophageal candidiasis and hairy leukoplakia are commonly described. Angular cheilitis, Kaposi's sarcoma and mycobacterial ulcers of the intestinal tract are less frequent manifestations.

Small intestinal coccidia, *Isospora belli* and *Cryptosporidium*, contribute to severe watery diarrhoea, malnutrition and weight loss and are commonly associated with the 'slim disease' of Uganda.

The HIV virus can produce enteropathic damage in the absence of an opportunistic infection.

There are no apparent interactions between HIV and helminths. There are as yet no significant reports of hyperinfection with *Strongyloides stercoralis* in AIDS.

Measles may be more severe in HIV-infected children and give rise to a significant enteropathy.

Salmonellosis is reported as being more common in AIDS patients.

Respiratory tract manifestations

Pneumocystis carinii pneumonia (PCP) is the commonest presentation of AIDS in America and Europe. In striking contrast PCP is rarely seen in Africa, and probably represents a geographical variation in the prevalence of *P. carinii*.

Tuberculosis is the main complicating respiratory infection in Africa, and appears to be due to reactivation of mycobacterial disease in patients with AIDS. HIV positivity is even higher in patients presenting with extrapulmonary tuberculosis, including lymphadenitis, meningitis, pleural and pericardial disease and miliary tuberculosis.

There is evidence to suggest that HIV-infected patients with pulmonary tuberculosis are less infective than HIV-negative patients. Pulmonary cavitation is less common and sputum smears for *M. tuberculosis* may be negative in a substantial number of patients with HIV infection and pulmonary tuberculosis. Developing countries, particularly in Africa, have reported marked increases in cases of tuberculosis associated with HIV infection. There is, therefore, concern that the population uninfected with HIV are being increasingly exposed to tuberculous infection.

To date infection with atypical mycobacteria has been rarely reported from Africa. There is evidence that in patients infected with both HIV and *M. leprae* there is accelerated progression of both diseases.

Central nervous system manifestations

The HIV virus and possibly cytomegalovirus cause encephalopathy and dementia in more than 50% of African AIDS patients. AIDS dementia is frequently accompanied by abnormal neurological signs including ataxia, neuropathy and myelopathy, and signs of loss of frontal lobe function.

Cerebral toxoplasmosis is probably a common but underdiagnosed complication of AIDS in Africa. Focal brain disease may also be due to cerebral lymphoma or tuberculoma.

Reactivation of tuberculosis may lead to the development of tuberculous meningitis. Cryptococcal meningitis is frequently observed in AIDS patients in Africa and reflects a high environmental exposure.

Progressive multifocal leukoencephalitis is found with increased frequency.

Retinitis may be caused by cytomegalovirus or toxoplasmosis.

Other protozoal infections in AIDS

HIV does not seem to impair immune responses to malaria at any stage of life including pregnancy, nor does malaria accelerate the course of HIV-related disease. The treatment of anaemia of malaria by blood transfusion is an important factor in the exposure of children to HIV.

HIV-seropositive subjects, with or without AIDS, have been reported with both new or recrudescent disease from infections with *Leishmania donovani*, *L. infantum* and *L. tropica*. Disease tends to be widespread in visceral leishmaniasis with cutaneous involvement.

No correlations have been made between HIV/AIDS and trypanosomiasis, nor with *Entamoeba histolytica*.

Other fungal infections in AIDS

The association with severe, often extensive, candidiasis has already been documented.

Infections with *Histoplasma capsulatum* appear particularly common in the Caribbean and central America, but not apparently in Africa, since the advent of AIDS.

Other miscellaneous conditions related to AIDS

Kaposi's sarcoma, an angioproliferative disorder of endothelial origin, presents in AIDS as a generalized aggressive disease with involvement of the skin, lymph nodes, lungs and gastrointestinal tract in particular.

Bacteraemia occurs more commonly in patients with AIDS. *Salmonella typhimurium* and *Streptococcus pneumoniae* are the most frequently isolated organisms in African patients.

Note. A discussion on the control of HIV/AIDS in the developing world is beyond the scope of this book. The reader is referred to Potts *et al.* (1991).

HUMAN T LYMPHOTROPHIC VIRUS 1

Human T lymphocyte 1 virus (HTLV-1) is an oncornavirus, that is an RNA tumour virus that can malignantly transform lymphocytes, and leads to neoplasia. The virus is endemic in South-west Japan and in parts of West and central Africa, in the black populations of the Caribbean, the southern states of the United States, and parts of South America. The virus is associated with two syndromes – adult T-cell leukaemia and lymphoma (ATLL) and tropical spastic paraparesis. Transmission occurs by routes similar to HIV, i.e. sexually and via blood and blood products, although ATLL has not yet been seen as a result of viral transmission by blood transfusion. Vertical transmission from mother to child through breast feeding appears an important route.

Patients with ATLL commonly have hepatosplenomegaly, generalized lymphadenopathy, lymphomatous meningitis and a variety of cutaneous lesions including generalized erythroderma and maculopapular rashes. Patients may suffer a rapidly progressive lethal illness, but subacute and smouldering forms are seen in at least one third of symptomatic patients. Pleomorphic leukaemic cells are found in the peripheral blood and eosinophils may be prominent. Lytic lesions are common in the skull and long bones and are associated with hypercalcaemia.

The lifetime risk of adult T-cell leukaemia developing after HTLV-1 infection is low, being in the order of 4% for patients infected before the age of 20.

Tropical spastic paraparesis (TSP) is a slowly progressive paraparesis affecting mainly the pyramidal tracts with minimal sensory deficit. TSP affects 10–100/100 000 of the population in tropical areas where HTLV-1 is endemic.

In the Caribbean HTLV-1 has also been associated with polymyositis, chronic relapsing infective dermatitis, and with increased susceptibility to strongyloidiasis.

A closely related virus, HTLV-II, originally isolated from two patients with hairy cell leukaemia, has recently been documented to occur in intravenous drug users. It has not yet been directly associated with any specific diseases.

26
Hepatitis

Acute hepatitis may result from a large number of viral and bacterial infections and reaction to drugs and chemicals (Table 26.1).

The hepatitis viruses (Table 26.2) share the potential for causing acute, and in some cases chronic, liver injury, but they are structurally and serologically unrelated.

Hepatitis A virus (HAV) is a worldwide community-acquired infection spread by the ingestion of water or food contaminated by human faeces. The virus is a picorna virus 27–32 μm in diameter. Chimpanzees, owl monkeys and marmosets are susceptible, but there is no evidence that they act as a reservoir of the virus for human disease.

Between 75 and 100% of the inhabitants of tropical countries have protective antibodies to HAV, acquired by inapparent or anicteric childhood infection. Fulminating infection is rare but can occur in pregnancy. In developed countries the fact that previously most adults had IgG antibodies to HAV was used as a basis for the preparation of normal immune (gamma) globulin (NIG) from pooled donor blood sera for use in short-term protection for tropical travel. In most developed countries now, however, improvements in hygiene have led to seropositivity rates in young adults of 10–15% or less, so that they are more susceptible to infection, and pooled serum is less useful for the production of passive immunity. In developed countries small epidemics of HAV hepatitis occur in schools, or may be related to the eating of infected shellfish.

HAV hepatitis is normally a mild inconvenient illness with a negligible mortality. After an incubation period of 3 to 4 weeks, the patient develops fever, muscle pains, nausea, anorexia, mild

238 Hepatitis

Table 26.1 Acute hepatitis – causes

Viruses	Bacterial infection	Chemicals	Drug reactions
Hepatitis A	Brucellosis	Mycotoxins	Isoniazid
Hepatitis B	Q Fever	Ethanol abuse	Rifampicin
Hepatitis C	Leptospirosis	Carbon tetrachloride	Sulphonamides
Hepatitis D	Typhoid	Paracetamol overdose	Phenothiazines
Hepatitis E	Pneumococcal pneumonia		Halothane
Yellow Fever	Pyomyositis		
Ebola/Marburg			
Cytomegalovirus			
Herpes simplex			
Coxsackie			
ECHO			

diarrhoea and right upper abdominal discomfort. Smokers lose the taste for tobacco.

After 3 to 4 days the fever and other symptoms subside as jaundice with bile-stained urine becomes apparent, and this remains for 1 to 2 weeks. Biochemical evidence of hepatitis has usually gone after about 4 weeks. It was thought that persistent infection with liver damage did not occur with HAV, but recent reports suggest that this may occur occasionally.

The diagnosis is suspected on clinical grounds. Liver function tests show marked rises in AST, ALT, GGT and conjugated bilirubin, and a modest rise in ALP. Leukopenia, with atypical lymphocytes present, is common. HAV antigen can be detected in the faeces at the onset of the clinical illness. HAV IgM antibodies are present in the acute illness and IgG antibodies after recovery.

Table 26.2 Hepatitis viruses

Type	Mode of spread	Disease Acute	Disease Chronic	Vaccine
A	Faecal–oral	+	?	Passive + active
B	Body fluids	+	++	Active + passive
C	Body fluids	+	++	–
D	Body fluids (with B)	+	++	–
E	Faecal–oral	++	–	–
F	Faecal–oral	++	–	–

Leptospirosis should be differentiated early in the illness; it is accompanied by marked muscle tenderness and polymorph leukocytosis. If the patient has recently travelled to the tropics malaria should be excluded.

There is no specific treatment for HAV hepatitis. Patients should rest, eat and recuperate as they wish. There is no evidence that enforced bed-rest, dietary changes or abstention from alcohol affect normal recovery.

Prevention of HAV infection depends on:

1. improved general hygiene, provision of toilets and washing of hands after defaecation, effective water and sewage treatments, purification of edible shellfish;
2. provision, for those lacking IgG antibodies, of NIG injections 0.02–0.12 ml/kg intramuscularly to provide protection for up to 4 months for tropical travel;
3. active vaccination with formalized whole virus by injection; members of communities with low herd immunity should be protected before tropical travel or perhaps before school entry.

Hepatitis B virus (HBV) infection is a worldwide but especially tropical disease of enormous importance because of its potential for causing chronic infection (in 200 million people), with risks of chronic active hepatitis, leading to cirrhosis, and, in some cases, hepatocellular carcinoma. The virus of HBV is a 42 μm particle (Dane particle) consisting of a core and a coat. It is a DNA virus containing three main antigens:

HBs Ag – surface antigen
HBc Ag – core antigen
HBe Ag – virulent antigen

to which antibodies are raised separately. A virulent mutant strain, recently discovered, lacks e antigen, however, and escapes protection by active vaccination.

HBV infection is transmitted by body fluids, e.g. blood, serum, sexual fluids. There are three epidemiological patterns:

1. In developed countries, spread occurs by exchange of blood or serum, especially through intravenous drug abuse, or by blood transfusion, by sexual intercourse, especially in prostitutes of either sex, and by invasive homosexual practices. Adult population rates of chronic carriage of HBs Ag vary from 0.1–5%.
2. In South-east Asia, 10–30% of the adult population are carriers

of HBs Ag, which is most often spread perinatally, with a 50% risk of infection in the baby of an infected mother.
3. In Africa, 5–15% of the adult population carry HBs Ag, which is usually spread via skin ulcers, needle sharing, tattoos, circumcision and ritual scarification during childhood and adolescence, and by sexual intercourse.

Chimpanzees, gibbons and orang-utan are susceptible but do not act as a natural reservoir for human transmission.

Infection with HBV may produce, after an incubation period averaging 12 weeks:

1. an acute hepatitis similar to that caused by HAV, but with a higher incidence of joint pains and rashes and other features of immune-complex deposition. Ninety per cent of cases recover fully and clear HBs Ag from the blood in 6 months, and HBe Ag in 3 months, and develop antibodies to core, then to e, then to s antigens.
2. chronic active hepatitis with persistent HBs antigenaemia, which is more virulent and potentially infective if HBe antigenaemia also persists. Antibodies to core but not to surface antigen are present. The activity of viral replication can be measured by the amount of HBV DNA polymerase in the blood. Chronic hepatitis results from the immune response to replicating virus incorporated into liver cell nuclei. Progression to cirrhosis and hepatocellular carcinoma is common.
3. 'silent' infection with low-grade chronic hepatitis which may nevertheless lead to cirrhosis and carcinoma.

The diagnosis of HBV infection is made by the demonstration of specific antigens and antibodies, interpreted in the light of evidence from liver function tests of active inflammation (raised AST, ALT, GGT) with DNA polymerase assay. The degree of liver damage is best assessed by the histological appearance of a liver biopsy. Alpha-foeto-protein levels in the blood give an indication of progression to carcinoma, which is otherwise diagnosed by ultrasonic scanning or computerized axial tomography, or by selective arteriography.

Acute HBV hepatitis requires no specific treatment. Corticosteroids should not be used, since they suppress the natural immune response and increase the risk of chronic infection. Chronic HBV hepatitis should likewise not be treated with corticosteroids. Various antiviral agents are under trial and many succeed in clearing HBs antigenaemia and controlling chronic inflammation, e.g. alpha-interferon, ribavirin, vidarabine. They are more likely to succeed if the chronic hepatitis is moderately active, as measured by AST, ALT and DNA polymerase levels. Success rates of up to 50% are possible, but the response is poor in Chinese and HIV-positive patients.

Patients should have regular measurements of serum alpha-foeto-protein. If hepato-cellular carcinoma is diagnosed early enough, partial hepatic resection may be successful; various chemotherapeutic regimens have also been employed, but most of the estimated 1 million deaths worldwide occur in people who receive no treatment.

There are two effective vaccines for active immunization against HBV infection, one derived from plasma and the other from recombinant virus infecting yeast cells. Both are expensive. In developed countries vaccination should be offered to all health care workers and those whose lifestyle puts them at special risk. In Africa the eventual aim is to immunize all children during their first year as part of their normal immunization programme. In the Far East vaccination needs to be started at birth in the infants of known carrier mothers and reinforced later.

Needlestick injury and other accidental injury with contaminated material should additionally be managed with HBV-specific immune globulin.

Other means of prevention include screening of blood donors, provision of sterile single-use needles and scalpels and education in safe sexual practices.

Hepatitis C virus (HCV) hepatitis is caused by a 50–60 μm RNA flavivirus, transmitted mainly by transfusion of blood and blood products, especially Factor VIII. Acute hepatitis occurs at an interval of 5 to 12 weeks; chronic hepatitis leading to cirrhosis and hepatocellular carcinoma is particularly important as it is thought to occur in at least 50% of those infected. HCV hepatitis occurs worldwide but is especially prevalent in southern Europe, the Middle East and Japan. Infection is also transmitted from mother to infant, by close domestic contact, and by sexual intercourse. Serological tests depend on the demonstration of anti-HCV antibodies by ELISA or PCR, and these should be employed in screening all donor blood. Chronic active HCV hepatitis can be treated with alpha-interferon or ribavirin.

Hepatitis D virus (HDV) occurs only in association with HBV and is a chimaera of HBs Ag coat and HDV Ag core, the latter being a virus similar to those causing hepatitis in woodchucks, ground squirrels, Peking ducks and herons. Combined B and D hepatitis can cause fulminating illness in intravenous drug abusers. A patient with chronic HBV hepatitis developing an acute exacerbation may have superadded HDV hepatitis. The two viruses may combine to cause chronic hepatitis with a high risk of cirrhosis and hepatocellular carcinoma. HDV is transmitted by body fluid exchange and is especially reported in southern Europe, the Middle East, India, tropical Africa and North and South America. Serological tests for HDV antigen and antibody are available.

Hepatitis E virus (HEV) hepatitis is a 27–34 μm RNA calicivirus, spread by the faecal-oral route, which causes epidemic hepatitis in young adults in the Indian sub-continent, central Asia, tropical Africa, Mexico and South-east Asia. The incubation period is 2 to 5 weeks. Acute hepatitis is similar to that caused by HAV, but there is a special risk, of up to 30%, of fulminating hepatitis and death in pregnant women. Chronic hepatitis does not appear to occur. An ELISA test for antibody is available.

Hepatitis F virus (HFV) hepatitis is the putative cause of acute fulminating community-acquired hepatitis not caused by any of the other known viruses; the virus has yet to be fully characterized.

27
Rabies

Rabies virus causes a fatal meningo-encephalitis in man, to whom it is transmitted by the bite or saliva of infected mammals, chiefly dogs, jackals, cats and bats, and rarely by human corneal grafting. The virus is a neurotropic RNA rhabdovirus; there are three similar viruses in Africa – Mokola, Duvenhage and Lagos bat – and a variant of Duvenhage virus in European bats has the potential to cause human disease. These viruses cause neuronal and ganglion cell death, with perivascular monocyte infiltration, throughout the brain, spinal cord and peripheral nerves. They spread up the axoplasm from the neurone nearest to site of entry and are then disseminated to all nerve tissue, including nerve endings in skin and cornea and exocrine organs, e.g. salivary glands. Characteristic Negri bodies are intra-cytoplasmic RNA inclusions especially found in the hippocampus, cerebellum and medulla.

The incubation period of human rabies is 20 to 60 days in most cases, but can extend up to 4 years. The shorter the distance from bite to brain the shorter the incubation. A prodromal illness of a few days of fever, restlessness and tingling or itching in the healed entry wound is usual. The patient then becomes agitated, reacting to noise and air movement with jerky muscle spasms, and hydrophobic; attempts to drink water are frustrated by severe facial muscle spasms ending in opisthotonos and convulsions. Excessive sweating and instability of blood pressure and body temperature are common.

Muscle paralysis may occur and be of either lower or upper motor neurone type. Males may suffer priapism. Delirium and coma presage death, which occurs within a few days. Human disease from the variant African viruses is identical.

Rabies

The differential diagnosis includes other types of viral encephalitis, organophosphate poisoning, tetanus, Guillain-Barré syndrome and phenothiazine dystonia. Laboratory diagnosis in the biting animal, if it can safely be caught, depends on immunofluorescence of brain tissue or demonstration of Negri bodies. In man, skin or corneal biopsy immunofluorescence is possible.

There is no effective treatment for rabies. Patients are extremely distressed and should be heavily sedated with chlorpromazine or opiates until death. Their saliva is infectious, and mouth-to-mouth resuscitation should not be attempted.

Several highly purified safe vaccines now exist:

HDCV (Merieux) human diploid cell
PVCV (Merieux) purified vero cell
PCECV (Behringwerke) purified chicken embryo cell

Pre-exposure immunization is given to those at special risk, e.g. veterinary and laboratory personnel, travellers to remote areas. HDCV 1ml i.m. is given initially, and 7 and 28 days later, and boosted 2-yearly. People at special occupational risk should have their antibody level checked 6-monthly.

Vaccination after exposure should be started as soon as possible, preferably within 24 hours.

HDCV 1ml i.m. is given on days 0, 3, 7, 14, 28 and 90. Various regimens using multiple intradermal doses are also used. In addition, human specific rabies immunoglobulin should be given in a dose of 20 iu/kg, half infiltrated into the wound, half into a distant muscle. Thorough cleansing of the wound with soapy water or alcohol or tincture of iodine will help to destroy the virus. Tetanus prophylaxis should also be given.

Rabies is especially common in tropical Africa and Asia, where dogs, jackals, monkeys and wolves are the commonest sources. In South America, vampire bats and dogs are the main reservoirs; in North America the risk is by spread from possums, skunks and raccoons, and in Europe from wild red foxes. Rabies is epizootic and transmitted to man in most countries of the world with the exception of islands such as Britain, Ireland, Cyprus, Australia, Borneo, New Guinea, Bali, New Zealand, Singapore, Japan, Taiwan and some of the Caribbean islands. Continental spread has yet to reach Spain, Portugal and Scandinavia (except for Denmark). Animal rabies has not existed in Britain since 1922, but 2000 cases yearly are confirmed in France, and over 5000 in Germany, and fox rabies occurs within 25 km of the channel ports. The cost of human post-exposure vaccination in France is 200 million Ffr annually and in USA 18 000 people each year are immunized, with a total cost of this and domestic animal protection estimated as 300 million US dollars.

Methods of prevention and control of rabies include:

1. control of dogs by shooting of strays, breeding limitation and vaccination of pet animals;
2. immunization of wild foxes with live attenuated oral vaccines in bait;
3. quarantine legislation for animals entering countries still free of disease;
4. immunization of farm animals;
5. health education.

Part Six
Fungal and Skin Diseases

28
Fungal Infections

Fungal infections of the skin flourish in tropical conditions. The scalp is infected by *Microsporum canis* to cause tinea capitis; oral griseofulvin for a prolonged period is the best treatment. Tinea corporis and cruris are caused by *M. canis* or *Trichophyton rubrum*. Systemic griseofulvin therapy can be enhanced by local application of an imidazole ointment. Chronic infection of the finger and toe nails due to *Tr. rubrum* (onychomycosis) also requires long-term griseofulvin.

Pityriasis versicolor, due to superficial infection with *Pityrosporon orbiculare*, is a common cause of patchy depigmentation in dark-skinned races, but also occurs in Caucasian skins. It must be distinguished from leprosy. Treatment is with oral griseofulvin and local application of selenium sulphide shampoo.

Mycetoma, in which a chronic deep-seated fungal infection causes tissue and bone destruction, usually in the foot, with chronic sinus formation, pain, deformity and disability, is a common problem in India, tropical Africa, the north of South America and Mexico, and is particularly difficult to treat. It may be caused by *Madurella mycetomatosis*, a true fungus with black spores, which may respond to prolonged treatment with ketoconazole or griseofulvin, or by *Streptomyces somaliensis*, an actinomycete with yellow spores, which is sensitive to streptomycin, dapsone and cotrimoxazole. In practice mycetoma is so destructive that some patients require amputation of the foot.

Other fungal infections entering the body through the skin include:

1. **chromoblastomycosis**, in which a variety of fungi cause verrucous papules, skin nodules and lymphoedema in tropical Africa and America. Treatment is difficult; thiabendazole and 5-fluocytosine are advocated.

2. **sporotrichosis**, due to *Sporothrix schenckii*, in Africa and tropical America, which starts with plaques and verrucous lesions but can spread to bones, lung and brain, especially in patients with AIDS. Itraconazole or amphotericin B are used in treatment.
3. **African histoplasmosis**, due to *Histoplasma duboisii*, in which skin papules and nodules can spread by lymphatics to invade bone. Ketoconazole, amphotericin B and cotrimoxazole have been used in treatment.

Cryptococcus neoformans has a major potential for causing meningo-encephalitis, but can also invade and damage bone and lung, especially in patients with AIDS. It is transmitted from the environment by inhalation. It can be stained in CSF by using Indian ink. Treatment is with ketoconazole or amphotericin B.

Inhaled fungi which cause primarily lung damage but can disseminate widely in the body include:

1. *Coccidiodes immitis* in the South-west USA, Mexico and South America, which presents with fever, cough, chest pain, cavitating lung lesions and pleural effusions, with eosinophilia, and is treated with ketoconazole, fluconazole or amphotericin B.
2. *Blastomyces dermatitidis* in tropical America, South USA, the Middle East and Africa which can produce skin nodules, ulcers and abscesses but also involve lung, bones, prostate and uterine cervix. Again ketoconazole or amphotericin B can be used in treatment.
3. *Histoplasma capsulatum* in southern USA which is a very common asymptomatic lung invader but causes destructive lung disease especially in AIDS patients and older males with cigarette-induced chronic airway disease. Ketoconazole and amphotericin B are useful treatments.
4. *Paracoccidiodes brasiliensis* in South America, especially Brazil, which can cause skin and bone lesions, lung damage and invasion of the liver, spleen, lymph nodes and bone marrow. Ketoconazole and amphotericin B are used in treatment.

In all these infections it is now possible, although very expensive, to use amphotericin B bound to liposomes; this markedly improves the therapeutic index of this effective, but toxic, fungicidal antibiotic.

Pneumocystis carinii was previously regarded as a protozoon but is now classified as a fungus. It is an ubiquitous human infection

Fungal infections

acquired by most inhabitants of tropical and temperate countries by inhalation in early childhood. It causes pneumonitis only in circumstances of immune suppression, e.g. AIDS, severe malnutrition, steroid and cytotoxic therapy and drug addiction. The symptoms are of progressive cough, dyspnoea and fever; chest radiographs may initially be normal, but subsequently perihilar shadowing gives way to diffuse nodular changes in mid- and lower lung zones. Definitive diagnosis rests with demonstration of the organism in sputum or in washings or biopsies obtained by bronchoscopy. *Pneumocystis carinii* pneumonia (PCP) is treated with high doses of cotrimoxazole or with pentamidine. Prophylaxis of further attacks in patients whose immunity remains compromised can be given with pentamidine by aerosol inhalation or oral dapsone with pyrimethamine ('Maloprim'), cotrimoxazole, or pyrimethamine with sulfadoxine ('Fansidar').

29
Skin Ulcers

Tropical skin ulcers are of three main types:

1. **Phagedenic ('tropical') ulcer.** This is caused by a mixture of beta-haemolytic streptococci, fusobacteria and spirochaetes, and occurs widely in the wet tropics, more in young males, usually below the knee. The ulcer is painful, moist and has a raised inflamed edge which is not undermined. It may complicate scabies mite infestation. Local treatment should consist of gentle regular toilet, avoiding removal of granulation tissue, and moist Eusol dressings. Systemic penicillin and metronidazole assist healing, as does rest of the leg if this is feasible. Chronic untreated ulcers spread widely over the leg, and may be complicated by squamous carcinoma.
2. **Cutaneous diphtheria** ('desert sore') occurs in dry hot climates, forming a painful sloughing ulcer with deeply undermined edges. Diphtheria toxin can cause paralysis in adjacent muscles but seldom affects distant muscles or myocardium. Treatment is with systemic penicillin and non-adherent dressings. Diphtheria antitoxin can be applied to the dressings or given by injection s.c. at an adjacent site.
3. **Buruli ulcer** due to *Mycobacterium ulcerans*, occurs in Africa, South-east Asia, Papua New Guinea and tropical America. It is painless but has a spreading undermined edge with skin bridges and satellite ulcers. It should be cleaned with silver nitrate and receive a skin graft after treatment with clofazimine, rifampicin or ofloxacin.

The differential diagnosis of these ulcerating diseases should include dracontiasis, lepromatous leprosy with neuropathic ulcer, skin tuberculosis ('lupus vulgaris'), cutaneous leishmaniasis, myiasis, syphilitic gumma, yaws and ischaemic ulcers in homozygous sickle-cell disease.

30
Myiasis

Myiasis is the presence of fly larvae in human tissue resulting from deposition of eggs by adult female flies. This occurs in necrotic tissue of open wounds or ulcers, in the nose or ear cavities, or in fistulae, and may be caused by a variety of flies:

Callitroga americana in tropical America
Chrysomya bezziana
Wohlfartia magnifica
Lucillia serilata } in Asia, Africa
Phormia regina
Musca domestica

Subcutaneous myiasis in healthy skin results in a painful papule which becomes an infested furuncle. Multiple lesions occur, and should be distinguished from impetigo, chicken pox and scabies. The dark spiracle of the larva (of *Dermatobia hominis* in tropical America, or *Cordylobia anthropophaga* in Africa) is visible in the centre of the lesion. Infection occurs when clothing is exposed to egg-laying female flies.

Wound and cavity myiasis is treated by careful debridement and instrumental removal of the larvae, and skin myiasis by suffocating the larvae by applying vaseline to the terminal spiracles, followed by removal.

Skin myiasis should be prevented by thorough ironing on both sides of washed clothes put outside to dry, to destroy fly eggs, or with drip-dry clothes, by drying them indoors in a fly-screened room.

Part Seven
Nutritional Diseases and Poisoning

31
Nutritional Deficiencies and Poisoning

PROTEIN ENERGY MALNUTRITION

Malnutrition in children in the tropics is important not only because it is common but also because it highlights important relationships between infection, immunity and nutrition which are of universal application.

All malnourished children show reduced growth and muscle protein synthesis, and have increased lipolysis with hypoglycaemia and hyperinsulinaemia. Where protein deficiency predominates, aldosterone secretion causes sodium and water retention, and growth hormone secretion is increased.

Two 'polar' types of protein energy malnutrition (PEM) are recognized – **marasmus** and **kwashiorkor**, but many children have a mixed clinical picture.

Marasmus occurs in infants aged under 1 year when maternal milk supply is interrupted by death or illness, and in older children in time of famine. The child has clearly lost muscle and subcutaneous fat. The skin is dry and wrinkled and there is no peripheral oedema. The hair is thin and dry. Body temperature is low. The child looks anxious but moves less than normal and may be hungry, but vomit any food offered. Such children are susceptible to diarrhoeal and respiratory infections, trachoma and vitamin A deficiency.

Children with kwashiorkor are usually aged 18 months to 4 years and have been weaned from the mother's breast. Muscle loss occurs but subcutaneous fat is preserved, and there is obvious peripheral oedema. The hair is dry, straight and depigmented. The skin is scaly and glistening, peeling and hyperpigmented, especially on the legs. The abdomen is distended and the liver enlarged. The child is fractious and irritable and often has diarrhoea. Clinical vitamin A deficiency may be present.

Children with mixed 'marasmic kwashiorkor' have a varied picture with muscle loss, oedema and damaged skin.

260 Nutritional deficiencies

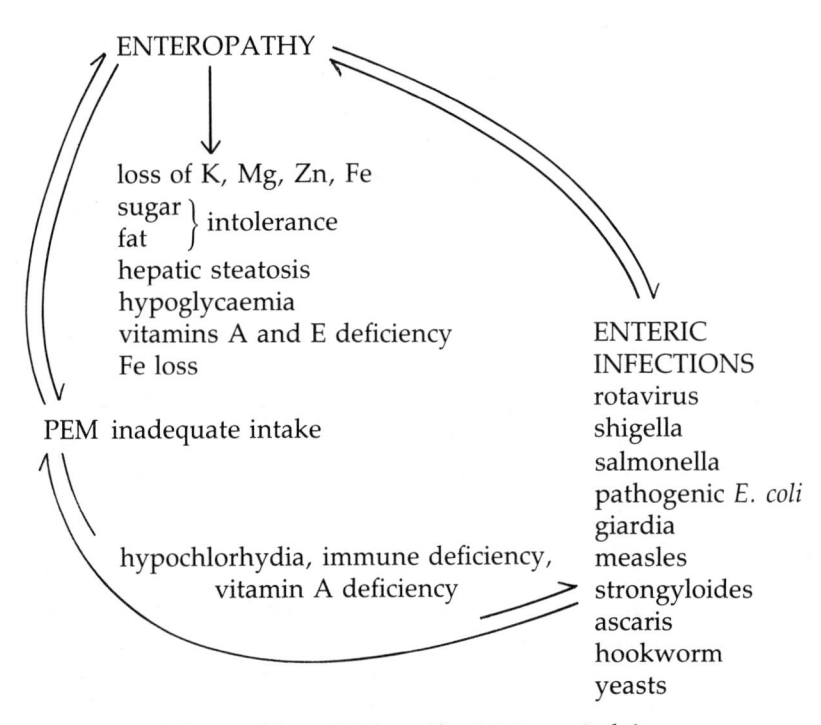

```
                ENTEROPATHY
                      │
                      ↓
        loss of K, Mg, Zn, Fe
        sugar ⎫
        fat   ⎬ intolerance
        hepatic steatosis
        hypoglycaemia
        vitamins A and E deficiency        ENTERIC
        Fe loss                            INFECTIONS
                                           rotavirus
  PEM  inadequate intake                   shigella
                                           salmonella
                                           pathogenic E. coli
                                           giardia
        hypochlorhydia, immune deficiency, measles
                 vitamin A deficiency      strongyloides
                                           ascaris
                                           hookworm
                                           yeasts
```

Fig. 31.1 Aetiology of kwashiokos: the 'vicious circle'

The pathogenesis of marasmus is usually simply that of reduced energy intake of whatever cause. The causes of kwashiorkor have been much debated and researched and are clearly multiple. The 'vicious circle' depicted in Figure 31.1 contains many responsible factors.

Reduced intake of protein, iron and vitamin A, and increased loss of zinc, have all been shown in childhood malnutrition to impair cellular immunity to infection, and the infections listed themselves aggravate the enteropathy. In addition it has been suggested that the response to infection mediated by interleukin 1 and tumour necrosis factor leads to an excess of free radicals (superoxide and hydrogen peroxide), which induces deficiency of glutathione, and is further aggravated by deficiencies of zinc, selenium, and vitamins A and E. A further factor in the causation of kwashiorkor is believed by some authorities to be the presence in many cereal weaning diets in tropical countries of excess amounts of aflatoxin and other fungal toxins, which are hepatotoxic and cytotoxic.

The diagnosis of the malnutrition syndromes is primarily clinical. Anthropometric documentation is essential for the individual child and for the study of the community. Body weight on a centile chart is a measure of current nutritional status, allowing for the presence of oedema; body length or height indicates previous progress in growth. Children with kwashiorkor have low serum albumin, potassium, zinc, magnesium and calcium levels and low blood sugar, and may be anaemic with defective blood clotting. Marasmic infants often have remarkably normal blood tests.

Clinical marasmus or kwashiorkor in older children and adults occurs in patients with AIDS with intestinal infections ('slim disease') and in abdominal and miliary tuberculosis.

The treatment of marasmus requires the provision of adequate nutrients appropriate to the age of the child, with powdered or cow's milk as the basis, involving the mother if possible at all stages.

The management of kwashiorkor is more complicated. Clinical dehydration at presentation should be treated with oral rehydration solution; intravenous fluids are best avoided as cardiac failure can easily be induced. Adequate intake of protein and calories requires frequent small feeds of a mixture of skimmed milk, vegetable oil and sugar (sucrose or glucose), followed by cereals, pulses, rice, eggs and meat or fish according to availability. Supplements of potassium and magnesium and vitamin A are important in early treatment, and should be followed with additional iron, folic acid and B vitamins. Stool and blood cultures and stool microscopy are essential; bacterial, helminthic and protozoal infections should be treated appropriately. Hypoglycaemic children can be given intravenous glucose but care is needed as this can induce or aggravate hypokalemia. If stools become unduly fatty on this feeding regimen, pancreatic extract can be added to the diet. Frothy acid stools imply intestinal hypolactasia and should lead to a reduction in lactose intake. Children with kwashiorkor may also have tuberculosis, and the diagnosis is made difficult by the impairment of cell-mediated immunity which causes negative skin tuberculin tests. Unexplained failure to thrive after correct initial treatment may justify a therapeutic trial of antituberculous therapy. Malaria may also complicate convalescence.

Prevention of childhood malnutrition in a community depends on:

1. adequate community food supplies;
2. education of mothers in the use of nutritious foods which are

cheap and available in their community, with eradication of superstitions such as the 'harmful' effects of foods containing protein (by causing 'heat');
3. primary health care programmes including monitoring of child development, treatment of or immunization against common infections, provision of vitamin A supplements.

VITAMIN A DEFICIENCY

Deficiency of retinol (vitamin A) affects 10 million children annually, of whom 1 million suffer permanent blindness, and is implicated in the impairment of immunity to many important infections. Preformed retinol is present in dietary liver, kidney, egg yolk and milk, and precusor carotenoids in green leafy vegetables and orange coloured vegetables and fruits.

Carotenoids are absorbed with fat in the small intestine and converted into retinol within the gut epithelial cell. Daily requirements are, in micrograms (retinol equivalents, REs),

children under 1 year	350
children 1–10 years	400
adults	600

Retinol is required physiologically for:

1. maintenance of epithelial integrity and mucus secretion;
2. sebum production in skin;
3. glycoprotein synthesis;
4. retinal photoreceptor cells (rhodopsin);
5. the efficiency of the immune system.

Serum retinol levels are reduced markedly in acute infections, especially measles, diarrhoea and respiratory tract infections.

The clinical effects of vitamin A deficiency are evident in the eye, in the following sequence:

1. impaired night vision;
2. xerosis (dryness) of the conjunctiva;
3. Bitot's spots – dry rough opaque patches in the conjunctiva of the temporal side of the eye;
4. keratomalacia and corneal ulceration;
5. opaque corneal scarring.

On the diagnosis of clinical vitamin A deficiency being made in a child, 100 000 REs should be given orally or i.m. at once and repeated on the next day, 14 days later, and again 3–4 months later. Children with measles should also be given 100 000–200 000 REs i.m. or orally during their illness; this has been shown to prevent eye damage and to reduce mortality, especially from respiratory infections.

Vitamin A deficiency in children occurs less in communities where breast-feeding is prolonged. Important dietary sources, to which the attention of mothers should be drawn, include red palm oil, carrots, mangoes, papayas, yellow sweet potatoes and dark green leafy vegetables. Egg yolk and fish liver oil are prime sources, and vitamin A can also be artificially added to bread, salt or sugar on a community basis.

BERI-BERI

Beri-beri results from deficiency of vitamin B_1 (thiamine) which is normally present in wholegrain rice, fish, meat, eggs and pulses. Deficiency states occur especially where rice is highly milled or over-boiled, and where carbohydrate forms a large proportion of energy intake, since thiamine is needed for its metabolism. Beri-beri occurs mainly in the poorer countries of South-east Asia, and can also be precipitated by alcohol if the diet is inadequate, in which case it may present as acute encephalopathy (Wernicke's). The clinical presentation may be predominantly neurological, with peripheral neuropathy, ataxia, confusion and tender muscles ('dry beri-beri'), or with cardiac failure ('wet beri-beri'). Infants of thiamine-deficient mothers present in the early weeks of life with restlessness, silent crying, vomiting, dyspnoea, tachycardia and hepatomegaly.

The clinical diagnosis is confirmed by a reduced red blood cell transketolase content.

Treatment in adults is with thiamine 100 mg i.v. and then oral supplements, and in infants with 25 mg i.v. and then supplementation by oral drops.

PELLAGRA

Pellagra occurs in populations who depend on maize as a food crop and who have a low dietary intake of animal protein. Nicotinic acid (niacin), a B vitamin essential for tissue respiration, is almost absent from maize. Pellagra is seen in Africa, the Middle East and Central India, and in alcoholics with a poor diet, but not in Central America where the staple tortilla, made from maize flour, has added lime juice which increases the availability of niacin. It is also seen occasionally in association with abdominal tuberculosis.

Clinically pellagra presents with anorexia, weakness, a painful burning tongue, dysphagia, diarrhoea, dermatitis (dark cracked rough skin in exposed areas), mental confusion and progressive dementia.

Treatment is with niacin (adults 100–200 mg t.i.d. children 10–12 mg t.i.d.).

RICKETS

Rickets and adult osteomalacia are caused by deficiency of vitamin D (cholecalciferol) which is formed by the action of ultraviolet light on skin containing 7-dehydrocholesterol derived from liver, eggs, butter, milk and fish oil in the diet. 25-hydroxy-vitamin D is then formed in the liver and converted in the kidney to 1:25-dihydroxy-vitamin D which, with parathormone, enhances intestinal absorption of calcium and phosphate and so is of primary importance in the development and integrity of the body skeleton. The daily dietary needs of vitamin D are 400 i.u. in infants, children, adolescents and pregnant women, and 200 i.u. in adults. Rickets in children causes softening of the skull bones and enlargement of long bone growth plates with deformity of the tibiae, ribs and other bones. In adults osteomalacia causes bone pain, fractures and loss of muscle bulk. In infants, vitamin D deficiency may present with hypocalcaemic tetanic convulsions and delayed tooth development.

Rickets occurs where the diet is deficient in the normal sources of vitamin D, but is also precipitated by lack of exposure to sunlight caused by 'purdah', voluminous clothing and dark overcrowded housing. A high dietary intake of phytate, e.g. in chapatti flour, also prevents vitamin D absorption. Rickets and osteomalacia also occur in intestinal malabsorption, chronic biliary obstruction, after gastrectomy, in chronic renal failure, and in patients on long-term anticonvulsant therapy.

Clinical rickets or osteomalacia is treated with 5000 i.u. daily of vitamin D or 1–3 μg daily of oral 1:25-dihydroxy-vitamin D. The most efficient method of community prevention is by appropriate fortification of baby milk formulae, cereals, milk, butter and chapatti flour with vitamin D, although excessive supplementation can cause harmful hypercalcaemia.

GOITRE AND CRETINISM

Endemic goitre and cretinism affect 200 million people, chiefly in mountainous areas of the developing world – the Himalayas, the Andes, Zaire, Central African Republic, Java, Papua New Guinea – where cooking salt is deficient in iodine, and potent sources of dietary iodine, such as egg yolk, spinach and kelp, are not available. In communities taking less than 40 mg of iodine daily endemic goitre occurs; if the intake is less than 20 mg daily most children have goitres, and cretinism occurs. Progressive adult goitre can cause pain (from bleeding into cysts) and, in extreme cases, respiratory embarrassment. Cretins may be 'myxoedematous' with markedly stunted growth and mental retardation, or 'nervous' with deaf-mutism, impaired growth, spasticity and mental retardation.

Preventive programmes should include:

1. injection of iodized oil i.m. in pregnancy;
2. iodination of salt.

ORGANOPHOSPHATE POISONING

Organophosphates are widely and increasingly used as insecticides in many tropical countries, and there are now many reports of accidental and suicidal poisoning by these highly toxic agents, which may be inhaled as vapour or penetrate intact skin or mucosae as liquid. 'Parathion' and 'malathion' are common causes of poisoning. It is estimated that up to 25 million episodes, 3 million of them serious, occur each year worldwide.

Poisoning with organophosphates can cause:

1. acute acetylcholinesterase inhibition, with bradycardia, miosis, increased secretion of tears, sweat and bronchial mucus, bronchospasm, muscle twitching, convulsions and rapid death;
2. sub-acute 'intermediate' syndrome, some 2–10 days after exposure, with muscle twitching and paralysis and compromise to respiration; this can occur even after correct treatment of acute poisoning;
3. in lower doses, chronic neuromyopathy and subtle dementia.

Acute poisoning requires urgent treatment with liberal doses of i.v. atropine, pralidoxime or obidoxime, and diazepam. Oxygen and artificial ventilation may be needed. Atropine dosage up to 100–200 mg may be needed over 48 hours. Intermediate syndrome may respond to further oxime treatment but ventilatory support may again be needed.

Special care is needed in agricultural communities where organophosphates are in use if metriphonate is to be given to control schistosomiasis, since this drug also has anticholinesterase effects.

TROPICAL ATAXIC NEUROPATHY

Ataxic neuropathy in the tropics may be caused by:

1. Nutritional deficiencies of **pyridoxine** or **pantothenic acid**. This occurs in Malaysia, Somalia, India and Jamaica and causes painful burning paraesthesiae in the legs, often with no evidence of peripheral neuropathy. It may be precipitated by isoniazid therapy in individuals who are slow acetylators of the drug. Treatment is with pyridoxine.
2. Thiamine deficiency (see beri-beri).
3. **Thiocyanate** toxicity, where cassava is the staple carbohydrate crop and is not stored or soaked to denature hydrogen cyanide. This results in sensory ataxia of the legs, deafness and optic atrophy. It may be alleviated by injections of vitamin B_{12} and supplements of thiamine and pyridoxine.

The differential diagnosis includes infection with HTLV-1, schistosomal transverse myelitis, spinal tuberculosis, alcoholism and lathyrism.

LATHYRISM

Lathyrism is an ataxic spastic paraplegia caused by the consumption, often as a 'famine crop', of certain species of legume (*Lathyrus sativus*, *L. cicera*, *L. chymenum*) which if not soaked thoroughly contain toxic amounts of beta-*N*-oxalylamino-alanine (BOAA), a non-protein amino acid. This disease occurs in India, where the offending food is called 'khesari dhal', and in Ethiopia and Algeria. Once spastic paraplegia has developed, there is no effective treatment.

32
Snake Bite

Poisoning by snake bite causes up to 30 000 deaths annually in India, is an important cause of death and morbidity in South-east Asia, Africa and tropical America, and also occurs in Europe, Australia and Papua New Guinea.

Rattlesnakes are common causes of poisoning in North America, *Bothrops* vipers in Central and South America. In Africa *Bitis* puff-adders and *Echis* saw-scaled vipers cause most poisoning, in the Middle East vipers and cobras, in Asia cobras, kraits and pit vipers. Australian land snakes cause poisoning in Australia and Papua New Guinea. Sea snake bites occur in all tropical waters.

Particular occupational risks of snake bite exist in rice farmers, cultivators of gardens, orchards and sugar-cane, fish farmers and sea fishermen, but snakes also often strike in peridomestic settings between dusk and human bed-time.

The toxic effects of snake families are, broadly:

1. vipers: tissue necrosis, shock, disturbed haemostasis, anaphylaxis;
2. elapids (cobras, kraits): muscle paralysis;
3. colubrids (keelback, boomslang, tree snakes): similar to vipers, but usually milder;
4. sea snakes: rhabdomyolysis.

Snake venoms are, however, complex mixtures of enzymes, polypeptides, amines and nucleotides; their clinical effects may vary within the same genus, and even in the same species in different countries. Thus rattlesnakes are also neurotoxic, some vipers are neurotoxic and do not affect haemostasis (e.g. Gaboon viper), the African spitting cobra causes local necrosis but not muscle paralysis, Australian land snakes cause rhabdomyolysis and disturbed haemostasis, and Russell's viper in Sri Lanka is neurotoxic whereas in India it usually is not. The South African berg adder is also neurotoxic.

Local swelling and tissue necrosis occur in most snake bites except those by kraits, coral snakes, sea snakes and most rattlesnakes. Early swelling may necessitate fasciotomy, and subsequent surgical debridement and skin grafting.

Disturbed haemostasis is a classical effect of viper bites; consumption coagulopathy results from endothelial damage, fibrin and platelet consumption, followed by enhanced fibrinolysis, and compounded by impaired platelet function. After several hours of delay a bleeding diathesis develops; this can be monitored by measurements of platelet count, serum FDP and fibrinogen levels, and whole blood clotting time. A serious complication may be acute anterior pituitary ischaemia, similar to Sheehan's syndrome, which requires steroid replacement therapy, with thyroid supplements later if the patient survives.

Acute cardiotoxicity may occur in the early syndrome of viper envenomation, but can be delayed for several days.

Acute renal failure complicates the bites of vipers, especially in India and Myanmar, sea snakes, and Australian land snakes, as a result of combination of direct toxicity, hypovolaemic shock, ischaemia, haemoglobinuria and myoglobinuria. Acute rhabdomyolysis is typically heralded by severe muscle pain ½ to 2 hours after envenomation, with evident myoglobinuria after some 2 further hours.

Muscle paralysis in elapid poisoning, and after the bites of other species mentioned above, may occur within minutes beginning in cranial nerve muscles and rapidly spreading to compromise respiration.

Asian cobras produce toxins which bind post-synaptically to acetylcholine at motor end plates, so that the clinical effects may respond to anticholinesterase treatment. Krait venom prevents acetylcholine release pre-synaptically, sometimes with a delay of several hours, and this does not respond to anticholinesterases.

The immediate management of snake bite is:

1. to reassure the victim that severe envenomation occurs in well below 50% of bites by most snakes;
2. to rest and immobilize the bitten part, usually a limb, as if fractured, to delay venom absorption;
3. to apply a large firm dressing just proximal to the bite site (not an arterial tourniquet);

4. to arrange transportation of the victim to hospital.

Where the snake is available and can safely be killed without serious damage to its head, it can be taken to the hospital for identification.

Active interference with the bite by suction, incision, freezing or even electrocution, is harmful or dangerous, and is likely to enhance venom absorption.

Hospital treatment is based on careful assessment of the patient to detect clinical effects of envenomation. An intravenous line should be established at once. For elapid bites with evidence of paralysis, treatment with anticholinesterases (neostigmine, with atropine) is given if an i.v. Tensilon test is positive; suitable antivenom should then be given in a dose of at least 100 ml i.v, (no less in children), with adrenaline and injectable antihistamines available to counter anaphylactic reactions. In serious cases artificial ventilation may be needed for some hours. Viper bite victims may suffer early shock, requiring i.v. resuscitation and hydrocortisone. Haemostatic defects are treated with infusions of blood, plasma, platelets or fibrinogen as needed, and as available, and with appropriate antivenom.

Tetanus immunoprophylaxis is essential. Antibiotic treatment may be needed to control infection in necrotic tissue, with possible surgical debridement and fasciotomy. If acute renal failure occurs this requires peritoneal dialysis.

Antivenoms used should be as specific to the snake as possible, and preferably made in the country in question from the local species.

In future it may be possible to utilize better knowledge of the content of snake venoms to provide monoclonal antibodies both for diagnosis of snake species and for treatment of poisoning.

The prevention of snake bite in tropical countries depends mainly on the education of the people in avoidance of risky locations and activities, and, where feasible, the wearing of protective clothing.

Part Eight
Eosinophilia and Unexplained Fever

33
Eosinophilia

Eosinophilia is commonly found in residents of and visitors to tropical countries, and in such circumstances usually implies an invasive helminthic infection, but it has many other allergic and non-infectious causes.

Eosinophilia is defined as an absolute eosinophil leukocyte count of over $0.45 \times 10^9/l$ and high eosinophilia as over $3.0 \times 10^9/l$, but the following causes of variability should be remembered:

1. There is a natural circadian rhythm with a peak at 24.00 hr and troughs at 08.00 and 18.00 hr.
2. In parasitic disease this diurnal variation may be exaggerated to cause changes of up to 200%.
3. African subjects appear to have a 'normal' eosinophil count of up to $0.8 \times 10^9/l$.
4. Immunosuppression, of whatever cause, abolishes the eosinophil reaction.
5. Adrenergic drugs increase, and adrenergic blocking drugs decrease, the eosinophil count.

Common helminthic causes of eosinophilia produce variable effects on the eosinophil count:

1. Marked eosinophilia in the invasive phase, then subsiding, occurs with schistosomiasis, strongyloidiasis, hookworm and ascariasis, especially in young children.
2. Sustained eosinophilia suggests trichinosis, toxocariasis or tropical (filarial) pulmonary eosinophilia.
3. Fluctuating eosinophilia occurs in dracontiasis, loiasis and filariasis.
4. Anatomically 'secluded' helminths, such as tapeworms, ascaris adults, biliary flukes and hydatid cysts may evoke no systemic eosinophilia.

Protozoal infections do not cause eosinophilia. Skin invasion by insects in scabies or myiasis can cause eosinophilia.

Assessment of the eosinophilic patient should start with a full history, with attention to travel details, insect exposure, diet, activities, animal contact and drug history. A full general examination should especially include a search for skin swellings or nodules, dermatitis, or evidence of moving larvae, for hydrocoele in males, for eye disease and for hepatosplenomegaly or jaundice.

Investigation of eosinophilia should start with a search for helminthic ova or larvae in stools, urine, sputum or duodenal juice as appropriate. Specific serological tests for most helminthic infections are now available; requests should be based on probabilities from the history and physical examination of the patient. Blood films at appropriate times should be examined for microfilariae, and skin snips taken if relevant. X-rays of chest, skull and deltoid area may yield useful information, and liver ultrasound can be used to demonstrate hydatid cysts. CT scanning of the head is a valuable tool in the assessment of cysticercosis.

If no evidence of helminthiasis is found, attention should be directed to 'non-tropical' causes of eosinophilia as follows:

1. **broncho-pulmonary allergy**, especially to aspergillus, for which a serological test is available;
2. **skin diseases**, e.g. urticaria, pemphigus, atopic eczema;
3. **drug allergy**, e.g. to sulphonamides, penicillins, cephalosporins, rifampicin, nitrofurantoin, isoniazid, phenothiazines, aspirin, phenytoin, quinidine, L-tryptophan;
4. **neoplastic diseases**, e.g. Hodgkin's disease, acute leukaemia;
5. **vasculitic/granulomatous diseases**, e.g. Wegener's granuloma, polyarteritis nodosa, Churg-Strauss syndrome. In this group of diseases various patterns of positive antineutrophil cytoplasmic antibody (ANCA) provide useful diagnostic information;
6. **'hypereosinophilic syndrome'** characterized by cardiomyopathy, neurological symptoms and thromboembolism;
7. **'eosinophilic gastroenteritis'** with abdominal pain and vomiting (*A. caninum* invasion of the small intestine should be excluded);
8. **variable eosinophilia** may occur in up to 10% of cases of tuberculosis, in sarcoidosis, in Addison's disease and scarlet fever.

In practice, a specific helminthic infection may be diagnosed and treated, or suspected and treated, empirically. In many visitors to the tropics eosinophilia may disappear on return to a temperate climate, either after empirical treatment (e.g. with albendazole, praziquantel or ivermectin) or after no treatment.

ANGIOSTRONGYLUS CANTONENSIS

In the Asian-Pacific region eosinophilic meningitis is caused by larvae of the rat lung-worm *Angiostrongylus cantonensis*, which has a life cycle involving snails, freshwater prawns and land-crabs as intermediate hosts. The patient has headache and neck stiffness with marked eosinophilia and a positive ELISA test. There is no satisfactory treatment; thiabendazole and similar drugs may aggravate the neurological syndrome by increasing the immune reaction to killed larvae. In severe cases, dexamethasone may be helpful to reduce this reaction. Most cases are eventually self-limiting.

34
Pyrexia of Unknown Origin

The investigation of fever in the tropics or after tropical travel should be based on the sequence:

1. a full and accurate history;
2. a careful clinical examination of the patient;
3. appropriate laboratory tests, X-rays and scans.

HISTORY

This should include residence and travel details, including the method and route of travel with any stopovers, and should allow for the possibility of exposure to insect vectors of tropical diseases in unusual circumstances, e.g. 'airport' and 'suitcase' malaria, or to disease transmitted by blood transfusion. Details of infectious human contacts, insect bite, animal contact, diet, occupation, activities and sports may all be relevant, and full documentation of prophylactic vaccinations and drugs should be obtained.

EXAMINATION

Specific attention should be directed towards:

Central nervous system

Altered consciousness or disturbed conjugate gaze may suggest cerebral malaria if full coma has not yet ensued. Delirium and drowsiness, sometimes with focal signs, may occur in typhus and typhoid fever. Neck stiffness suggests meningitis or encephalitis, but meningism can occur in many fevers, including leptospirosis and malaria. African trypanosomiasis may cause an acute brain syndrome in early Rhodesian cases, and progressive dementia in the Gambian form. HIV-related infections of the CNS include cryptococcal meningitis and cerebral toxoplasmosis.

Skin

Many tropical fevers cause rashes or other skin lesions:

1. **Macular rash** occurs in typhus, typhoid, dengue and other arbovirus infections, secondary syphilis, measles, early HIV seroconversion illness, Epstein-Barr virus infections.
2. **Haemorrhagic rash** occurs in yellow fever and other viral haemorrhagic fevers, relapsing fever, leptospirosis, meningococcal and gonococcal septicaemia, Rocky Mountain spotted fever.
3. **Other skin lesions** include circinate erythema in early trypanosomiasis, erythema migrans in Lyme disease, the eschars of scrub and Mediterranean and African tick-borne typhus and of cutaneous anthrax, and the facial rash of systemic lupus erythematosus. Leprosy reaction states are accompanied by fever.

Joints

Tropical fevers which can cause arthritis, affecting a few or many joints, include Lyme disease, melioidosis, fungus infections, relapsing fever, brucellosis, rubella, tuberculosis, Reiter's syndrome after genital or intestinal infections, salmonellosis, Yersiniosis and many arbovirus infections.

Throat

Exudative pharyngitis occurs especially in streptococcal infections, Epstein-Barr virus infection, Lassa fever and diphtheria, and should be distinguished from oropharyngeal candidiasis, which commonly occurs in AIDS.

Lungs

Clinical evidence of pneumonitis or pleural disease can occur in many infections which are common in the tropics, including:

Streptococcus pneumoniae
Mycoplasma pneumoniae

Haemophilus influenzae
Legionella pneumophila
Chlamydia psittaci
Pneumocystis carinii (although this is less common in AIDS patients in the tropics)
Tuberculosis – miliary, pulmonary, postpulmonary, pleural
Fungus infections
Pneumonic plague or anthrax
ARDS due to *P. falciparum* malaria
Toxoplasmosis
Q Fever
Typhus
Typhoid
Entamoeba histolytica – especially right basal signs
Tropical pulmonary eosinophilia

Heart

Acute rheumatic fever is common in the tropics, as is bacterial endocarditis complicating congenital and rheumatic heart disease. Endocarditis with negative cultures for common organisms may be caused by Q fever or brucellosis. Acute pericarditis may be viral, but a virulent tuberculous form occurs in AIDS patients.

Lymph nodes

Many tropical fevers cause lymphadenopathy but, if it is marked, possibilities include visceral leishmaniasis, infection with Epstein-Barr virus, HIV or cytomegalovirus, tuberculosis, trypanosomiasis, toxoplasmosis, typhus (especially scrub), and the local bubo of plague.

Hepatosplenomegaly

This also occurs in many tropical fevers, notably malaria and typhoid, but if marked, should lead to consideration of visceral leishmaniasis, Q fever, brucellosis, lymphomas and chronic myeloid leukaemia, and Katayama syndrome.

Other localizing signs

These include those of spinal tuberculosis (with possible psoas abscess), tropical pyomyositis, amoebic liver abscess, osteomyelitis and dental, nasal sinus, and ear infections.

Fever without physical signs

Without early laboratory evidence of a diagnosis (e.g. malaria, typhoid), this may suggest miliary tuberculosis, a deep-seated abscess or tumour, systemic lupus erythematosus, polyarteritis nodosa, sarcoidosis or a drug reaction.

Abdominal signs and symptoms

These may vary from constipation in early typhoid and typhus through diarrhoea in gut infections, *P. falciparum* malaria, visceral leishmaniasis and Katayama syndrome to severe pain in leptospirosis, sickle-cell crisis, spinal or abdominal tuberculosis, amoebic liver abscess, or 'spontaneous' bacterial peritonitis in hepatic cirrhosis and nephrotic syndrome.

Where no other clinical clues are present, the simple laboratory test of a differential white blood cell count gives helpful information.

	Fever under 2 weeks	*Fever over 2 weeks*
PNL high	Pus, septicaemia Leptospirosis Relapsing fever Collagen disease	Pus, amoebic liver abscess
PNL normal	–	Trypanosomiasis, TB, brucellosis, syphilis, toxoplasmosis
PNL low	Viruses Rickettsiae Typhoid Miliary TB	Miliary TB, visceral leishmaniasis, brucellosis

(PNL Polymorphonuclear leukocyte count)

INVESTIGATION PLAN FOR FEVER AFTER TROPICAL EXPOSURE

Full blood count
Chest X-ray
Malaria blood smears (3–6 sets)

Investigation plan for fever

Culture urine, stool, blood, bone marrow
Bone marrow stained for TB, visceral leishmaniasis
Stool and urine microscopy for parasite ova or larvae
Serology appropriate to history and clinical findings
Ultrasound liver, kidneys
Intravenous urography
Liver biopsy
Spleen puncture for visceral leishmaniasis
Dental X-ray, spinal X-ray
Gallium or indium scanning
LE cells

In some clinical situations a delay in diagnosis to await full confirmation may be dangerous and firm proof may be difficult to achieve. A therapeutic trial of suitable drug(s) may be appropriate, e.g. quinine in suspected *P. falciparum* malaria, antituberculous drugs in suspected miliary, abdominal or pericardial TB and doxycycline in suspected typhus.

Part Nine
Travelling to the Tropics

35
Outlines of Immunization and Protection of the Traveller

International travel, including visits to the developing world, is increasing for both business and leisure pursuits. This chapter will attempt to provide the rationale to determine which immunizations, prophylactic medications and other preventive measures are appropriate for travellers to the tropics and subtropics.

IMMUNIZATIONS

Poliomyelitis

One hundred and seventy-five cases of paralytic poliomyelitis were imported into industrialized countries between 1975 and 1984. Of these 47 were in holiday travellers, spending often no longer than a week overseas.

No adult should remain unimmunized against poliomyelitis. Individuals born in the UK before 1958 may not have been immunized and no opportunity should be missed to immunize them in adult life. A course of three doses of oral poliomyelitis vaccine (OPV) is recommended for the primary immunization of adults. A reinforcing dose should be offered to people travelling outside of Europe, North America, Australia and New Zealand. For those exposed to a continuing risk of infection, a single reinforcing dose is desirable every 10 years.

OPV should not be given during the first trimester of pregnancy, unless there is a definite risk of polio. Immunization should be postponed in the light of a febrile illness or diarrhoea and vomiting, and is contraindicated for the immunosuppressed. OPV may be given at the same time as any other vaccine. If not given simultaneously with other live virus vaccines, an interval of 3 weeks should be observed. The effect of OPV is inhibited if given less than 3 weeks before or within 3 months after an injection of normal immunoglobulin.

Typhoid

Typhoid vaccination may be offered to travellers to Africa, Asia and Latin America, particularly when travelling outside the usual tourist areas. It is especially recommended for travel to the Indian sub-continent where the risk of typhoid has been estimated to be 120 per 1 million travellers each week to India and Pakistan.

Inactivated monovalent typhoid vaccine is 70–90% effective for 3–7 years. Primary vaccination is 0.5 ml subcutaneously followed 4 weeks later by 0.1 ml intradermally. Booster doses of 0.1 ml intradermally may be given every 3 years. A single primary dose gives less complete protection but may be adequate for short duration travel. The uptake of vaccine is diminished by the high incidence of side-effects when the subcutaneous route is used. Travellers can be inconvenienced or incapacitated by local pain and swelling. Repeated injections of typhoid vaccine increase the risk of hypersensitivity.

A single dose modified Vi capsular polysaccharide vaccine, which is less reactogenic, has recently been licensed for use in the UK. Antibody seroconversion is observed in over 90% of recipients after administration of a single dose. In young children antibody responses may be sub-optimal.

Ty21a, an attenuated strain of *Salmonella typhi* that lacks the Vi polysaccharide, has been developed as a live oral vaccine, given on alternate days for 3 to 4 doses. The liquid formulation gives superior protection to the enteric coated capsular formulation.

The safety of the monovalent killed vaccine, the Vi capsular polysaccharide vaccine, and the live attenuated Ty21a oral vaccine has been demonstrated in pregnancy. Their use in pregnancy should reflect the actual risk of disease and probable benefits of the vaccine.

Cholera

Currently available cholera vaccines, whether prepared from Classic or El Tor strains, are of limited usefulness, and the risk to most international travellers is so low that it is questionable whether vaccination is of any benefit. Vaccines have been shown to provide only about 50% effectiveness in reducing the incidence of clinical illness for a period of 3–6 months. They do not prevent transmission of infection.

The World Health Organization and International Health Regulations no longer recommend cholera vaccination for travel to or from cholera-infected areas. Some countries, however, still sometimes require evidence of cholera vaccination for entry. Complete primary immunization consists of two doses of vaccine given 1 week to 1 month or more apart,

When travellers visit areas where cholera is prevalent, and are likely to cross borders from such areas, particularly overland, they should be advised to have the vaccine before travel, and carry a valid certificate of vaccination, rather than risk injections abroad. One injection is sufficient.

Prevention of cholera is by close attention to personal and food hygiene. Only treated water should be drunk. Food should be cooked thoroughly and eaten hot. Shellfish should be avoided in affected areas and raw fruit and vegetables should only be eaten if they can be peeled.

Hepatitis A prophylaxis

Hepatitis A affects about 1 in 500 travellers to the tropics who are not protected by immune globulin. The risk of acquiring hepatitis A by persons travelling abroad varies with living conditions, length of stay and the incidence of hepatitis A in the area visited. Immune globulin is generally recommended for travellers to developing countries if they will be eating in settings of poor sanitation or will be visiting extensively with local persons, especially young children.

For persons who might require repeated immunoglobulin prophylaxis, screening for anti-hepatitis A antibodies before travel may be useful to define susceptibility and eliminate unnecessary prophylaxis for those who are immune.

The response to live attenuated vaccine viruses may be diminished if given concurrently with immunoglobulin. In general, parenterally administered live vaccines should not be given for at least 6 weeks after immunoglobulin administration. Immunoglobulin does not, however, interfere with immune responses to yellow fever vaccine.

A candidate vaccine against hepatitis A will shortly be available. Studies with inactivated vaccines in large numbers of human volunteers have shown that these vaccines are safe, induce high seroconversion rates with two doses given 1 month apart, and induce neutralizing antibodies at concentrations that usually exceed the peak concentration after one dose of human normal immunoglobulin. A third dose results in higher concentrations of antibody which should provide long-term protection.

Hepatitis B

Hepatitis B vaccination should be considered for persons, health care workers in particular, who plan to reside for greater than 6 months in areas with high levels of endemic hepatitis B, and who will have the types of contact with the local population that are likely to transmit hepatitis B infection. An excessive risk of hepatitis B is associated with sexual promiscuity.

Japanese encephalitis

In temperate areas transmission occurs in late summer and autumn. This includes areas such as China and Japan, and the northern areas of Bangladesh, Myanmar, India, Cambodia, Laos, Vietnam, Thailand and Nepal. In subtropical and tropical areas, such as south India, Malaysia, Indonesia, Philippines, Sri Lanka, Taiwan and south Thailand, the risk of transmission is present throughout the year, but it is accentuated during the rainy season and early dry season, when the mosquito population is highest.

The risk of Japanese encephalitis to short-term travellers and persons who confine their travel to urban areas is low. Travel in rural areas where rice culture and pig farming are common increases the risk. Prevention is important because the case-fatality rate is over 25% and the risk of serious neurological sequelae is high.

Two doses of formalin inactivated Japanese encephalitis vaccine ('Biken vaccine'), given 1–2 weeks apart, are necessary to protect against disease. The vaccine does not afford full protection until 1 month after the second dose. A booster dose after 1 year will provide extended protection.

Meningococcus

Regular epidemics of meningococcal A disease occur in sub-Saharan Africa, India, Nepal and Saudi Arabia. A quadrivalent polysaccharide vaccine is available against groups A, C, Y and W135, and is recommended for travellers to the meningitis belt of Africa and to these other areas when outbreaks are present.

Vaccination is not recommended during pregnancy unless risk of infection is substantial. The vaccine gives a poor response in infants, particularly those under 18 months of age.

Primary vaccination for both adults and children is a single 0.5 ml dose of vaccine administered subcutaneously, and gives 2–3 years of protection.

Rabies

Pre-exposure vaccination with human diploid cell rabies vaccine (HDCV), an inactivated virus vaccine, should be considered for travellers who will be living in, or long-term visitors to, countries where rabies is a constant threat. Pre-exposure vaccination does not eliminate the need for additional therapy after a rabies exposure but simplifies post-exposure treatment by eliminating the need for rabies immune globulin and by decreasing the number of post-exposure doses of vaccine required.

A booster immunization or measurement of antibody levels should be performed every 2 years for those at continuing risk. Chloroquine, taken for malaria prophylaxis, may interfere with the response to rabies vaccination.

BCG vaccine

This is advisable for tuberculin negative individuals intending to live or travel for prolonged periods in countries where tuberculosis is endemic.

Yellow fever

Yellow fever vaccine is a live, attenuated virus preparation. Persons 9 months of age or older who are travelling in rural areas of South America or Africa where yellow fever is officially reported should be vaccinated. Vaccination should also be considered for travel outside urban areas of countries which do not officially report the disease, but which lie in the yellow fever endemic zone. Yellow fever vaccination and a valid certificate of vaccination is required by some countries if a person is arriving from or has travelled through a yellow fever endemic zone.

A single dose of 0.5 ml is given irrespective of age. The International Certificate is valid for 10 years from the tenth day of primary vaccination and immediately after revaccination. Yellow fever vaccine is only given at centres approved by the WHO.

Pregnant women, because of the theoretical risk of foetal infection, should not be vaccinated, unless the risk of yellow fever outweighs that of vaccination. It is contraindicated in the immunosuppressed, and should not be given to either symptomatic or asymptomatic HIV-positive individuals since there is as yet insufficient evidence as to the safety of its use.

If one or more live vaccines are required, they should be given at the same time in different sites or with an interval of 3 weeks between them.

Tetanus

Tetanus is more common in developing countries. The risk of developing tetanus is only increased in those with increased risk of exposure, e.g. agricultural workers. Provided a full primary course has been previously completed, the normal overseas traveller does not require a tetanus booster.

INTERNATIONAL TRAVEL, SEXUALLY TRANSMITTED DISEASES AND HIV

Often insufficient attention is paid to the risks of acquiring sexually transmitted diseases and HIV infection through heterosexual intercourse during foreign travel.

People behave differently when they travel. Tourists travel to seek adventure and new experiences, including sex. The importance of travellers in the transmission of sexually transmitted diseases (STDs) is demonstrated by the rapid worldwide spread of penicillinase-producing strains of *N. gonorrhoeae* (PPNG). In western countries up to 30% of new cases of syphilis are found to be acquired abroad.

Despite most travellers being knowledgeable about sexual transmission of HIV there is often no perceived risk of HIV infection associated with travel. All organizations concerned with travel need to increase education about HIV/AIDS and make all travellers more aware of the risks of acquiring HIV infection while abroad. Health care providers giving advice to travellers need to be able to discuss sensitive issues, such as sexual behaviour, openly in clear and easily understood language, and should take every opportunity to do so.

The risk of travellers acquiring HIV infection from infected needles or blood is greater in areas where HIV is prevalent and routine screening of blood for HIV antibodies has not been fully established. This increased risk can be minimized by seeking health care facilities where such screening is done routinely, and by not sharing needles.

TRAVELLER'S DIARRHOEA

Visitors to the tropics and subtropics are at considerable risk of developing a diarrhoeal illness, with attack rates of 30–50% in those who travel to the developing world. Numerous studies have assessed the many bacterial, parasitic and viral pathogens associated with traveller's diarrhoea. In most studies, enterotoxigenic *Escherichia coli* (ETEC) has been the most commonly isolated pathogen, accounting for up to 70% of cases.

ETEC infection produces a self-limiting diarrhoea lasting 4–7 days. Associated cramping abdominal pain is common.

Prevention

Antimicrobial drugs such as neomycin, doxycyline, quinolone antibiotics, co-trimoxazole and trimethoprim, when taken prophylactically, reduce the frequency of traveller's diarrhoea. However, the risks of antimicrobial prophylaxis include allergy, rash, photosensitivity, blood dyscrasias, Stevens-Johnson syndrome, staining of teeth in children, and promotion of other infections such as antibiotic-associated colitis and candidal vaginitis. Widespread use of antimicrobial drugs for chemoprophylaxis cannot therefore be recommended. A case may be made for the use of quinolone antibiotics, to which resistance is not yet an apparent problem, when it is vital that the visitor to an endemic area must perform with maximum efficiency.

An alternative approach to prophylaxis, popular in North America, is the use of bismuth subsalicylate. In a rather high dose of 60 ml or 2 tablets (524 mg) four times daily, protection rates of about 65% have been achieved, by a mechanism which is not entirely clear. Its use gives rise to a black tongue and black stools and is contraindicated if the person is allergic to salicylates.

The heat-labile toxin produced by ETEC is closely related in structure and immunological determinants to cholera toxin. A combined cholera toxin B subunit/whole cholera vaccine, whilst showing itself to be useful in the prevention of cholera, is also able to reduce diarrhoea due to heat-labile toxin producing ETEC by more than 60%. A vaccine against ETEC may therefore be on the horizon.

Recent work on a mouse model suggests that exposure to certain *Lactobacilli* species can diminish the subsequent ability of *E. coli* to colonize the stomach and small intestine. Such an approach may find application in the protection of travellers against diarrhoea.

Treatment

The prevention and treatment of dehydration and acidosis is the cornerstone of management of acute watery diarrhoea from all causes. Oral administration of glucose-electrolyte solutions is effective for promoting water and sodium absorption and correcting acidosis.

The role of antibiotics in the treatment of acute watery diarrhoea is limited. Antimicrobials including co-trimoxazole, trimethoprim, doxycycline and the 4-fluoroquinolones are effective in diminishing the duration of the diarrhoea and increasing clearance of the pathogen. The arguments against using antibiotics for treatment are much the same as those given for reserving their use in prophylaxis. Under some circumstances judicious treatment with a quinolone antibiotic may be appropriate.

Symptomatic treatment with antidiarrhoeal drugs such as diphenoxylate or loperamide should never be used as an alternative to oral rehydration therapy, should not be used in infants and young children because of the risk of respiratory depression, and should not be used if an invasive pathogen, e.g. *Shigella*, is suspected.

PREVENTION OF MALARIA

Malaria prevention and chemoprophylaxis has been covered in Chapter 1.

HEAT ILLNESS

The health hazard posed by high environmental temperature and humidity is frequently underestimated. In hot climates, particularly after physical exercise, sweating may lead to excessive loss of salt and water. An increased fluid intake is necessary. The loss of excess salt can be countered by the addition of extra table salt to meals. Within 2 weeks the sweating mechanisms adapt to the climatic conditions with a reduction in both the volume and salt concentration of sweat. The maintenance of adequate hydration, however, remains important but normal salt intake can be resumed.

Heat injury, variously named as 'heat stroke' or 'heat-exercise hyperpyrexia', is caused by failure of the normal heat dissipation mechanisms allowing an excessive rise in core temperature. Failure of adequate heat transfer to the environment is usually due to high environmental temperature or humidity, although other factors such as excessive clothing and lack of air movement are important. Other factors predisposing to heat illness are vigorous exercise, age, poor acclimatization, alcohol abuse, obesity, febrile illness, heart disease, drugs (especially anticholinergics, diuretics and phenothiazines) and inadequate fluid intake.

The early manifestations of heat-exercise hyperpyrexia include nausea, dizziness, confusion, inco-ordination and irritability. There may be rapid development of circulatory failure, hypoxia, metabolic acidosis, disseminated intravascular coagulation, myoglobinuria and renal failure.

Rapid reduction of core temperature is the cornerstone of treatment. This can be achieved by tepid sponging of the exposed body surface accompanied by vigorous fanning. Fluid replacement should follow as soon as possible.

Bibliography

Chapter 1

Chulay, J.D. and Ockenhouse, C.F. (1990) 'Host receptors for malaria – infected erythrocytes'. *Am. J. Trop. Med. Hyg.*, **43**(2), Suppl., 6–14.

Clark, I.A., Chaudhuri, G. and Cowden, W.B. (1989) 'Roles of tumour necrosis factor in the illness and pathology of malaria'. *Trans. R. Soc. Trop. Med. Hyg.*, **83**, 436–40.

Malaria Reference Laboratory and the Ross Institute. (1989) 'Prophylaxis against malaria for travellers from the United Kingdom'. *Br. Med. J.*, **299**, 1087–9.

Mitchell, G.H. (1990) 'Progress toward malaria vaccination'. *Curr. Opin. Infect. Dis.*, **3**, 387–92.

Newton, C.R.J.C., Kirkham, F.J., Winstanley, P.A. *et al.* (1991) 'Increased intracranial pressure in Kenyan children with cerebral malaria'. *Lancet*, **337**, 573–6.

Waller, D., Crawley, J., Nosten, F. *et al.* (1991) 'Intracranial pressure in childhood cerebral malaria'. *Trans. R. Soc. Trop. Med. Hyg.*, **85**, 362–4.

Warrell, D.A., White, N.J., Veall, N. *et al.* (1989) 'Cerebral anaerobic glycolysis and reduced cerebral oxygen transport in cerebral malaria'. *Lancet*, **ii**, 534–8.

Warrell, D.A., Molyneux, M.E. and Beales, P.F. (eds) (1990) 'Severe and complicated malaria', 2nd edn, WHO. *Trans. R. Soc. Trop. Med. Hyg.*, **84**, Suppl. 2, 1–65.

Wernsdorfer, W.H. and McGregor, I. (1988) *Malaria – Principles and Practice of Malariology*, Churchill Livingstone, Edinburgh.

Chapter 2

Badaro, R., Falcoft, E., Badaro, F.S. *et al.* (1990) 'Treatment of visceral leishmaniasis with pentavalent antimony and interferon gamma'. *N. Engl. J. Med.*, **322**, 16–21. (Illustrates recent treatment trials.)

Chulay, J.D., Bhatt, S.M., Mugai, R. *et al.* (1983) 'A comparison of three dosage regimens of sodium stibogluconate in the treatment of visceral leishmaniasis in Kenya'. *J. Infect. Dis.*, **148**, 148–55. (This provides food for thought on the differing sodium stibogluconate treatment regimens.)

Chunge, C.N., Ouate, J., Pamba, H.O. *et al.* (1990) 'Treatment of visceral leishmaniasis in Kenya by aminosidine alone or combined with sodium stibogluconate'. *Trans. R. Soc. Trop. Med. Hyg.*, **84**, 221–5. (Illustrates recent treatment trials.)

Peters, W. and Killick-Kendrick, R. (eds) (1987) *The Leishmaniases in Biology and Medicine*, 2 volumes, Academic Press, London. (The most up-to-date comprehensive volume on leishmaniasis – a source book.)

Playfair, J.H.L., Blackwell, J.M., Miller, H.R.P. *et al.* (1990) 'Modern vaccines: Parasitic diseases'. *Lancet*, **335**, 1263–6. (Includes a review of leishmanial immunology and vaccine developments.)

Singh, M.P., Mishra, M., Khan, A.B. *et al.* (1989) 'Gold treatment for kala-azar'. *Br. Med. J.*, **299**, 1318. (Illustrates recent treatment trials.)

Thakur, C.P., Kumar, M. and Kumar, P. (1988) 'Rationalisation of regimens of treatment of kala-azar with sodium stibogluconate in India: a randomised study'. *Br. Med. J.*, **296**, 1557–61. (This provides food for thought on the differing sodium stibogluconate treatment regimes.)

Chapter 3

Griffiths, W.A.D. (1987) 'Old World cutaneous leishmaniasis', in *The Leishmaniases in Biology and Medicine*, Volume 2, (eds W. Peters and R. Killick-Kendrich), Academic Press, London, 617–36.

Walton, B.C. (1987) 'American cutaneous and mucocutaneous leishmaniasis', in *The Leishmaniases in Biology and Medicine*, Volume 2, (eds W. Peters and R. Killick-Kendrich), Academic Press, London, 637–64.

Chapter 4

Haller, L., Adams, H., Merouze, F. *et al.* (1986) 'Clinical and pathological aspects of human African trypanosomiasis (*T.b.*

gambiense) with particular reference to arsenical encephalopathy'. *Am. J. Trop. Med. Hyg.*, **35**, 94–9.

Molyneux, D.H., de Raadt, P., Seed, J.R. *et al.* (1984) 'African human trypanosomiasis', in *Recent Advances in Tropical Medicine*, Vol. 1, (ed H.M. Gilles), pp. 39–62.

Pepin, J. Milford, F., Guern, C. *et al.* (1987) 'Difluoromethylornithine for arseno-resistant *Trypanosoma brucei gambiense* sleeping sickness'. *Lancet*, **ii**, 1431–3.

Van Miervenne, N. and LeRay, D. (1985) 'Diagnosis of African and American trypanosomiasis'. *Br. Med. Bull.*, **41**, 156–61.

World Health Organization. (1986) Epidemiology and control of African trypanosomiasis. Report of a WHO Expert Committee, Geneva. WHO. Tech. Rep. Ser. 1986 (No. 739).

Chapter 5

de Rezende, J.M. and Moriera H. (1988) 'Chagasic megaoesophagus and megacolon. Historical review and present concepts'. *Arq. Gastroenterol.*, **25**, 32–43.

Gutteridge, W.E. (1985) 'Existing chemotherapy and its limitations'. *Br. Med. Bull.*, **41**, 162–8.

Hudson, L. and Britten, V. (1985) 'Immune response to South American trypanosomiasis and its relationship to Chagas' disease'. *Br. Med. Bull.*, **41**, 175–80.

Luquetti, A.O., Miles, M.A., Rassi, A. *et al.* (1986) '*Trypanosoma cruzi*: zymodemes associated with acute and chronic Chagas' disease in central Brazil'. *Trans. R. Soc. Trop. Med. Hyg.*, **80**, 462–70.

Oliveira, J.S.M. (1985) 'A natural human model of intrinsic heart nervous system denervation: Chagas' cardiopathy'. *Am. Heart. J.*, **110**, 1092–7.

Schofield, C.J. (1985) 'Control of Chagas' disease vectors'. *Br. Med. Bull.*, **41**, 187–94.

Chapter 6

Guerrant, R.L. (1986) 'Amebiasis: introduction, current status, and research questions'. *Rev. Infect. Dis.*, **8**, 218–27.

Sharma, M.P., Rai, R.R., Acharya, S.K. *et al.* (1989) 'Needle aspiration of amoebic liver abscess'. *Br. Med. J.*, **299**, 1308–9.

Walsh, J.A. (1986) 'Problems in recognition and diagnosis of amebiasis: estimation of the gobal magnitude of morbidity and mortality'. *Rev. Infect. Dis.*, **8**, 228–38.

Chapter 7

Farthing, M.J.G. (1989a) 'Host–parasite interactions in human giardiasis'. *Q. J. Med.*, **70**, 191–204.
Farthing, M.J.G. (1989b) *'Giardia lamblia'*, in *Enteric Infection: Mechanisms, Manifestations and Management*, (eds M.J.G. Farthing and G.T. Keusch), Chapman and Hall Medical, London, pp. 397–413.

Chapter 8

Mata, L. (1986) *'Cryptosporidium* and other protozoa in diarrheal disease in less developed countries'. *Pediatr. Infect. Dis. J.*, **5**, S117–S130.

Chapter 9

Cook, G.C. (1991) 'Antihelminthic agents: some recent developments and their clinical application'. *Postgrad. Med. J.*, **67**, 16–22.

Chapter 10

Case Records of the Massachusetts General Hospital (Case 20-1990) (1990) *N. Engl. J. Med.*, **322**, 1446–58. (A discussion of the differential diagnosis of neurocysticercosis.)
Cook, G.C. (1988) 'Neurocysticercosis: parasitology, clinical presentation, diagnosis, and recent advances in management'. *Q.J. Med.*, **68**, 575–83.
Horton, R.J. (1989) 'Chemotherapy of *Echinococcus* infection in man with albendazole'. *Trans. R. Soc. Trop. Med. Hyg.*, **83**, 97–102.

Chapter 12

Case Records of the Massachussets General Hospital (Case 33-1990) (1990) *N. Engl. J. Med.*, **323**, 467–75. (The differential diagnosis of a case of hepatic clonorchiasis.)
Singh, T.S., Mutum, S.S. and Razaque, M.A. (1986) 'Pulmonary paragonimiasis: clinical features, diagnosis and treatment of 39 cases in Manipur'. *Trans. R. Soc. Trop. Med. Hyg.*, **80**, 967–71.
Strauss, W.G. (1962) 'Clinical manifestations of clonorchiasis. A controlled study of 105 cases'. *Am. J. Trop. Med. Hyg.*, **11**, 625–30.

Chapter 13

Allen, M.B. and Cooke, N.J. (1991) 'Corticosteroids and tuberculosis.' *Br. Med. J.*, **303**; 871–2.

British Thoracic Society. (1985) 'Short-course chemotherapy for tuberculosis of lymph nodes: a controlled trial'. *Br. Med. J.*, **290**, 1106–8.

Elliot, A.M., Luo, N., Tembo, G. et al. (1990) 'Impact of HIV on tuberculosis in Zambia: a cross sectional study'. *Br. Med. J.*, **301**, 412–5.

Fox, W. (1988) 'Tuberculosis case-finding and treatment programmes in the developing countries'. *Br. Med. Bull.*, **44**, 717–37.

Harries, A.D. (1990) 'Tuberculosis and human immunodeficiency virus infection in developing countries'. *Lancet*, **i**, 387–90.

Parsons, M. (1989) 'The treatment of tuberculous meningitis'. *Tubercle*, **70**, 79–82.

Pettengell, K.E., Larsen, C., Garb, M. et al. (1990) 'Gastrointestinal tuberculosis in patients with pulmonary tuberculosis'. *Q. J. Med.* **275**, 303–8.

Strang, J.I.G., Gibson, D.G., Mitchison, D.A. et al. (1988) 'Controlled clinical trial of complete open surgical drainage and of prednisolone in treatment of tuberculous pericardial effusion in Transkei'. *Lancet*, **ii**, 759–64.

Chapter 15

Watt, G., Padre, L.P., Tuazon, M.L. et al. (1988) 'Placebo-controlled trial of intravenous penicillin for severe and late leptospirosis'. *Lancet*, **i**, 433–5.

Chapter 16

Meningitis – Future Challenges. (1991) Proceedings of a Symposium organized by USNMRU3 and the Royal Society of Tropical Medicine and Hygiene. *Trans. R. Soc. Trop. Med. Hyg.*, **85** (suppl. 1); 1–47.

Chapter 19

World Health Organization. Simplified approaches for sexually transmitted disease (STD) control at the primary health care level. Report of a WHO Working Group. WHO/VDT/85.437, Geneva.

World Health Organization. STD treatment strategies. Report of a WHO Working Group. WHO/VDT/89.447, Geneva.

Chapter 22

Brown, G.W., Robinson, D.M., Huxsoll, D.L. et al. (1976) 'Scrub typhus: a common cause of illness in indigenous populations'. *Trans. R. Soc. Trop. Med. Hyg.*, **70**, 444–8.

Hart, R.J.C. (1991) 'Chronic Q fever,' in *Current Topics in Clinical Virology*, (ed P. Morgan-Capner), Public Health Laboratory Service, London.

Helmick, C.G., Bernard, K.W. and D'Angelo, L.J. (1984) 'Rocky Mountain spotted fever: clinical, laboratory, and epidemiological features of 262 cases'. *J. Infect. Dis.*, **150**, 480–8.

Maeda, K., Markowitz, N., Hawley, R.C. et al. (1987) 'Human infection with *Ehrlichia canis*, a leukocytic rickettsia'. *N. Engl. J. Med.*, **316**, 853–6.

World Health Organization Working Group on Rickettsial diseases. (1982) Rickettsioses: A continuing disease problem. *Bull. WHO*, **60**, 157–64.

Chapter 23

Baird-Parker, A.C. (1990) 'Foodborne salmonellosis'. *Lancet*, **336**, 1231–5.

Blacklow, N.R. and Greenberg, H.B. (1991) 'Viral gastroenteritis'. *N. Engl. J. Med.*, **325**, 252–64.

Blaser, M.J. and Reller, L.B. (1981) '*Campylobacter* enteritis'. *N. Engl. J. Med.*, **305**, 1444–52.

Case Records of the Massachusetts General Hospital (Case 15-1990) (1990) *N. Engl. J. Med.*, **322**, 1067–75. (A case of tropical sprue with a discussion of the differential diagnosis.)

Clemens, J.D., Sack, D.A., Harris, J.R. et al. (1990) 'Field trial of oral cholera vaccines in Bangladesh: results from three-year follow-up'. *Lancet*, **335**, 270–3.

Clemens, J.D., Van Loon, F., Sack, D.A. et al. (1991) 'Biotype as determinant of natural immunising effect of cholera'. *Lancet*, **337**, 883–4.

Cohen, J.I., Bartlett, J.A. and Corey, G.R. (1987) 'Extra-intestinal manifestations of salmonella infections'. *Medicine*, **66**, 349–87.

Cook, G.C. (1984) 'Aetiology and pathogenesis of postinfective tropical malabsorption (tropical sprue)'. *Lancet*, **i**, 721–3.

Cover, T.L. and Aber, R.C. (1989) '*Yersinia enterocolitica*'. *N. Engl. J. Med.*, **321**, 16–24.

Gilks, C.F., Brindle, R.J., Otieno, L.S. et al. (1990) 'Life-threatening bacteraemia in HIV-1 seropositive adults admitted to hospital in Nairobi, Kenya'. *Lancet*, **336**, 545–9. (*Salmonella typhimurium* is an important cause of morbidity and mortality.)

Glass, R.I., Claeson, M., Blake, P.A. *et al.* (1991) 'Cholera in Africa: lessons on transmission and control for Latin America'. *Lancet*, **338**, 791–5.

Keusch, G.T. and Bennish, M.L. (1989) 'Shigellosis: recent progress, persisting problems and research issues'. *Pediatr. Infect. Dis. J.*, **8**, 713–19.

Chapter 25

Potts, M., Anderson, R. and Boily, M.-C. (1991) 'Slowing the spread of human immunodeficiency virus in developing countries'. *Lancet*, **338**, 608–13.

(1990) 'Parasitic and other infections in AIDS', *Trans. R. Soc. Trop. Med. Hyg.*, **84** (Suppl. 1), 1–39.

Chapter 34

Harries, A.O., Myers, B., Battacharrya, D. *et al.* (1986) Eosinophilia in Caucasians returning from the tropics. *Trans. R. Soc. Trop. Med. Hyg.*, **80**, 327–8.

Spry, C.J.F. (1980) Eosinophilia and hypereosinophilic syndromes. *Trans. R. Soc. Trop. Med. Hyg.*, **74** (Suppl.), 3–6.

Chapter 35

Cossar, J.H. and Reid, D. (1989) 'Health hazards of international travel'. *World Health Stat. Q.* **42**, 61–9.

Dickinson, J.G. (1989) 'Heat-exercise hyperpyrexia'. *J. R. Army Med. Corps.*, **135**, 27–9.

Farthing, M.J.G. (1991) 'Review article: prevention and treatment of traveller's diarrhoea'. *Aliment. Pharmacol. Therap.*, **5**, 15–30.

Walker, E. and Williams, G. (1989) *ABC of Healthy Travel*, 3rd Edn, British Medical Journal.

World Health Organization (1992) *International Travel and Health. Vaccination Requirements and Health Advice*, WHO, Geneva.

Index

Page numbers underlined refer to differential diagnosis.
Italicized numbers refer to tables.

Abdominal tuberculosis 138–141
Abscess
  'collar stud' (amoebic dysentery) 57
  lung 186
  paraspinal <u>145</u>
  psoas 143
  skin 186
Achlorhydria 67
Acyclovir 179
Adrenergic blocking 273
Aedes mosquito 223, 225
AIDS (Acquired Immunodeficiency Syndrome) <u>43</u>, 231–5, 291
  abdominal tuberculosis 138
  CNS involvement 233–4
  cutaneous manifestation 232
  diarrhoea 73
  fungal infection 234
  giardiasis 67
  heterosexual spread 231
  intestinal infection 232–3
  malnutrition 261
  meningoencephalitis 250
  protozoal infection 234
  pyrexia 278
  respiratory tract infection 233
  strongyloidiasis 83
  tuberculosis 147–48
  see also HIV; Immunosuppression
ALA, *see* Amoebic liver abscess
Albendazole 81–2, 85, 86, 87, 88, 98, 99
Albuminuria 224
Alcoholism <u>266</u>
Allergic eosinophilia 273

Allergic response, and onchocerciasis 106–7, 108
Alopecia, leishmaniasis 26
Alpha-interferon 241
Amodiaquine 15, 20
Amoebiasis 55–65
  aetiology 55–6
  anogenital 60
  carriers 61, 65
  clinical features 56–60
  control 65
  diagnosis 60–3
  faecal transmission 55–6
  treatment 63–5
Amoebic dysentery 56–8, 60–2, 64
  carriers 61
  treatment 64
  see also Amoebiasis
Amoebic liver abscess (ALA) 58–60, 62, 65, <u>170</u>
Amoebic serology 62–3
Amoeboma 58, 64
  see also Amoebiasis
Amoxycillin 170, 181
Ampicillin resistance 166
Anaemia
  acute haemolytic 13
  iron deficiency 81, 82
  leishmaniasis 26
  malarial 6, 8, 16
Ancylostoma duodenale, *see* Hookworms
Angiostrongylus cantonensis 275
Anorexia, in shigellosis 214
Anthrax <u>43</u>, 187–88
Antibiotics, *see specific drug*

304 Index

Anticholinesterase 268
Antigenic variation 40
Antimony, in leishmaniasis 28, 37
Appendicitis <u>58</u>, <u>183</u>, <u>216</u>
Arbovirus <u>11</u>, <u>196</u>, 223–30, 278
Artemisinine 15
Arthralgia 201
Arthritis 106, 164
Ascariasis 77–80
Ascaris lumbricoides 77
  see also Ascariasis
Ascites 137, 139, 140
Ataxic neuropathy 266
ATLL (adult T cell leukaemia and lymphoma) 235
Atropine 265

Bacillus anthracis 187
Back pain 143
Bacteraemia 162, 234
BCG vaccination 134
Benznidiazole 52
Beri beri 263, 266
Biken vaccine 288
Bilharzia, see Schistosomiasis
Biliary obstruction 78
Black fly 107
Bladder wall fibrosis 112–13
Blastomyces dermatitidis 250
Blindness 144–5
  see also Onchocerciasis
Boil, staphylococcal <u>187</u>
Bone destruction 249
Bone marrow, granulomas in 185
Bone softening 264
Borrelia spp. 158, 159
Boutonneuse fever *192*, 194
Bowel perforation 57
Brain abscess 65
Breast feeding 49, 265
Brill-Zinsser disease 191, 195
British Thoracic Society tuberculosis regimen 132–3
Brucellosis <u>43</u>, <u>170</u>, 185–6, <u>188</u>, <u>200</u>, 238, 278, 279
Brugia spp., see Filariasis
Bubo 176, 178, 279
Bubonic plague 188–9
Buruli ulcer <u>109</u>, 253

Calabar swellings 105, 106
Calymmatobacterium granulomatis 179
Campylobacter enteritis 216–17
Candida albicans 180, 181–2
Candidal balanitis 182
Candidiasis 181–2, 234, 278
Capillary stasis 6
Carcinoma
  colon <u>58</u>
  spine <u>143</u>
Cardiac failure, in kwashiorkor 261
Cardiomyopathy 50, 105
Cardiotoxicity, viper bite 268
Carrier
  cholera 206
  meningococcal meningitis 161
Cartilage destruction 35
Cassava 266
Ceftriaxone 178, 181, 183
Cercarial dermatitis 112, 113
Cerebral cysticercosis 92, 92–3
Cerebral oedema 94
Cerebral paragonimiasis 124–5
Cerebral tuberculomas <u>93–4</u>
Cestodes, see Tapeworms
Chagas' disease, see Trypanosomiasis, American
Chagoma 50, 51
Chancre, trypanosomal 42
Chancroid 176
Chicken pox <u>255</u>
Chiclero's ulcer 32–3, *33*
  see also Leishmaniasis, cutaneous
Chikungunya 224, 226
Chlamydia trachomatis 177–8
Chlamydial conjunctivitis 183
Chloramphenicol 163, 166, 167, 168, 170, 197–8
Chloroquine 12, 13, 14–15, 17, 19
  and rabies vaccine 289
Cholangitis 115
Cholera 205–8
  vaccine 286–7
Chromoblastomycosis 249
Ciprofloxacin 171, 181
Cirrhosis 241, 242
Clofazimine 153
Clonorchis sinensis 115–7
Clostridium perfringens 212–13

Clostridium tetani 173
Clotrimazole 182
CNS
  AIDS 233–4
  fever 277–8
  trypanosomiasis 42, 43–4
  typhoid 170
Coccidiodes immitis 250
Colic, ureteric 142
Colitis
  shigellosis 213
  ulcerative 61
Colonic stricture 57
Coma, malarial 8, 9
Combantrin 79, 82
Congo-Crimea haemorrhagic fever 224, 229
Conjunctivitis, neonatal 183
Constipation 51, 280
Cord compression 143, 144
Corticosteroids
  cerebral malaria 16
  hepatitis B 239
  loiasis 105
  TBM 147
Cotrimoxazole 170
Coxiella burneti 200
Coxsackie *238*
Cretinism 265
Crohn's disease 139
Cryptococcous neoformans 250
Cryptosporidiosis 73–4
Cutaneous larva migrans 82–3
Cutaneous manifestations of AIDS 232
Cutter vaccine 189
Cysticercosis 92, 92–3, 227
Cystitis 142, 183
Cytomegalovirus 200, *240*

Dapsone 151
DCL (diffuse cutaneous leishmaniasis) 33, *35*, 37
Deafness 169, 195
DEC, *see* Diethylcarbamazine
Dehydration 207
  see also Oral rehydration
Dengue 163, *224*, 225–6, 278
Dermatitis 84, 112, 113

Desert sore 253
Dexamethasone 125, 164
Diarrhoea 280
  acute watery 205–3
    cholera 205–8
    Clostridium perfringens 212–13
    E. coli 210–11
    salmonellosis 209–10
    vibrio parhaemolyticus 209
  AIDS-related tuberculosis 147
  chronic 217–19
  cryptosporidiosis 73–4
  dysenteric 213–17
    E. coli 215–16, 216–17
    shigellosis 213–15
    Yersinia enterocolitica 217
  giardiasis 68
  malarial 7
  mucous 121
  schistosomiasis 112, 113
  traveller's 291–2
  trichinosis 86
  typhoid 169
Diethylcarbamazine (DEC) 88, 104, 105
Diloxanide furoate (furamide) 64, 65
Diphtheria 278
Diphtheria toxin 253
Dogs as reservoirs of infection
  fluke 114
  hydatid disease 95, 97
  leishmaniasis 24, 25, 32
Downgrading reaction 151, 153
Doxycycline 20, 157, 177, 208, 291
Dracontiasis 108–9, 253, 273
Dracunculus medinensis, 101, 108–9
Drug resistance
  ampicillin 166
  P. falciparum 12–13, 14–15
  sulphonamides 163, 164
D-xylose excretion 70
Dysentery 213–17
  see also amoebic dysentery; diarrhoea
Dysphagia 139
Dyspnoea, in tuberculosis 137
Dysuria 142, 180

Ebola fever 229, *238*

ECG in pericardial tuberculosis 137
Echinococcus granulosus 95–8
Echinococcus multilocularis 98–9
Echinostomiasis 122
Eclampsia 11
Ectopic fluke migration 118, 124–5
Eflornithine (DFMO) 45
Ehrlichiosis 200–1
El Tor cholera 208
Elephantiasis 103, 104
Emetine hydrochloride 63–4
Empyema 132
Encephalitis 92, 174, 243–4, 277
  from arboviruses 224, 226–28
  herpes virus 226–7
  tick-borne 228
  viral 11
  and vitamin B_1 deficiency 263
Encephalopathy 105, 233–4
Endocarditis 170, 185, 199, 201, 279
Entamoeba histolytica 55–6
  see also Amoebiasis
Enteric (typhoid) fever 169–71
Enteritis, necrotizing 212, 212–13
Enterohaemorrhagic *E. coli* (EHEC) 215–16
Enteroinvasive *E. coli* (EIEC) 216
Enteropathogenic *E. coli* (EPEC) 211
Enterotoxigenic *E. coli* (ETEC) 207, 210–11, 291–2
Eosinophilia 84, 86, 97, 273–5, 279
Epileptic seizure 145
Epithelioma 36
Epstein-Barr virus 185, 200, 278, 279
Erythema nodosum leprosum 151, 152–3
Erythromycin 64, 159, 176, 181
Eschar 195, 196
Escherichia coli 210–11, 215–16
Espundia 35–6, 37
Ethambutol 133, 136, 141
Eye damage by onchocerciasis 107
Eye, toxicity of ethambutol 131

Facioliasis 117–18
Faeces
  amoebiasis 55–6
  ascariasis 79

cryptosporidiosis 73
as fertilizer 77
giardiasis 68
Fansidar 20
Fasciolopsis buski 118–19
Fever 5, 26, 163, 277–81
  see also Enteric fever; Relapsing fever; Rickettsioses
Filariasis 101, 103, 103–5, 273
Fistula 139, 178
Fits 92
Flea-borne infection 188–89
Fluke
  ectopic migration 118, 124–5
  intestinal 118–22
  liver 114–18
  lung 122–5
  see also Schistosomiasis
Francisella tularensis 188
Fungal infection 186, 234, 249–51, 278, 279
Furamide (diloxanide furoate) 64, 65

Gall bladder 169, 209
Gammaglobulin elevation 27–8
Ganglion loss, Chagas' disease 51
Gangrene, of typhus 195
Gas, intestinal 68
Gastrodisciasis 121–2
Gastrointestinal bleeding 139
Genital tuberculosis 142
Genital ulcer 175–80
Genitourinary tuberculosis 141–2
Giardia lamblia 67–8, 69
  see also Giardiasis
Giardiasis 67–71
Glossina spp., see Tsetse fly
Goitre 265
Gonorrhoea 180–1, 183
Granuloma formation 185
Granuloma inguinale 179
Granuloma multiforme *152*
Granulomata, in tuberculosis 130
Griseofulvin 249
Guinea worm 108–9

Haematuria 142
Haemolytic-uraemic syndrome 215–16

Haemophilus meningitis 165–7
Haemophilus influenzae 161, 165–7
Haemophilus ducreyi 176
Haemoptysis 96–7
Haemorrhagic fevers 224, 228–30
Halofantrine 15, 20
Halzoun 118
'Hanging groin' 107
Hantaan virus 230
Heat stroke 11, 293
Helminthic infection 274, 275
Hepatic malignancy 62
Hepatitis 238
   A 237–39
   A/B prophylaxis 287–88
   alpha-interferon 241
   B *238*, 239–41
   C *238*, 241
   D *238*, 241–2
   E/F *238*, 242
   Q fever 199
   trypanosomal 50
   viral 11, 170, 224
Hepatocellular carcinoma 239, 240
Hepatomegaly, in tuberculosis 137
Hepatosplenomegaly 26, 158, 235, 279
Herpes 178–79, 232, *238*
Heterophyiasis 120
Histoplasma capsulatum 250
Histoplasmosis 250
HIV (Human Immunodeficiency Virus) 175, 210, 231, 290–1
   see also AIDS
Hookworms 78, 79, 80–3
   non-human 82–3
Human T lymphotrophic virus 1 (HTLV 1) 235, 266
Hydatid disease 62, 95–9
   cyst removal 97–8
   metastases 96–7, 99
Hydrocephalus 92, 146–7
Hydronephrosis 142
Hydrophobia 243
Hyperinfection syndrome 84, 85
Hypernephroma 97
Hyperoesinophilic syndrome 274
Hyperparasitaemia 17

Hypersensitivity, in tuberculosis 130
Hypertension, intracranial 94, 124, 145
Hypnozoites (*Plasmodia* spp.) 4, 5
Hypogammaglobulinaemia 67
Hypoglycaemia 6, 11, 16
Hypopigmentation 149, 150, 249
Hypotension 9, 16, 111, 137

Ileitis 169
Ileo-caecal tuberculosis 139
Ileum, cryptosporidiosis in 73
Immune complexes in meningitis 164
Immune response, in schistosomiasis 111, 112
Immune system, and retinol 262
Immune tolerance 103
Immunity, and malnutrition 260
Immunity to drugs, *see* Drug resistance
Immunization, *see* Vaccine
Immunoperoxidase test 197
Immunosuppression 273, 285
   see also AIDS
Impetigo 255
Inferior mesenteric vein, flukes in 111, 113
Influenza 11
Intestinal infection of AIDS 232–3
Intestinal obstruction 78, 79, 213
Intestinal perforation 57, 169
Intracranial pressure, raised 94, 124, 145
Intussusception 78
Iodine deficiency 265
Iritis 150
Isoniazid 133, 136, 138, 141, 146, *238*
Ivermectin 104, 108
IVM, *see* Divermectin

Jacksonian fits 92
Jarisch-Herxheimer reaction 159
Jaundice 238
Jejunum, hookworms in 80

Kala-azar, *see* Leishmaniasis
Kanamycin 183
Kaposi's sarcoma *152*, 232, 234

Katayama syndrome 86, 112, 113, 279
Keloid 152
Kerandel's sign 42
Keratitis 107, 150
Khesari dhal 266
Kwashiorkor 259, 260, 261
Kyphosis 143

Lactase deficiency 70
Larva currens 84
Larva migrans 82–3, 88, 109
Laryngitis, tuberculous 132
Lassa fever 224, 228, 278
Lathyrism 266
Legionellosis 200
Legumes, and lathyrism 266
Leishman-Donovan (LD) bodies 37
Leishmania spp. 24, 25
Leishmaniasis
　cutaneous 31–8, 152, 253
　　clinical features 34–6
　　DCL 33, 35
　　diagnosis 36–7
　　epidemiology 31–2
　　immunity 34
　　localized 34–5
　　pathology 32–4
　　reservoirs 25, 32
　　therapy 37–8
　mucocutaneous 33, 35
　　espundia 35–6
　visceral 23–9, 43, 279
　　clinical features 26–8
　　epidemiology 23–5
　　prevention 29
　　treatment 28–9
Leishmaniasis recidiva 33, 35, 36
Leishmanin skin test 28, 33–4
Leprosy 33, 149–53
　differential diagnosis 27, 36, 109, 152, 255
Leptospira spp. 155
Leptospirosis 11, 155–7, 196, 200, 224, 238, 278
Leukaemia 26, 235, 274
Leukopenia 201
Levamisole 79
Lichen planus/simplex 152

Liver
　abscess, *see* Ameobic liver abscess
　enlarged 59, 112
　granulomas in 185
　hydatids 96, 99
Liver function tests 11, 62
Loa loa 102, 105, 109
Loeffler's pneumonitis 78
Loiasis 105–6, 273
Louse-borne
　relapsing fever 158
　typhus 191–2, 194–5
Lung abscess 124, 186
Lung flukes 122–3, 124–5
Lung hydatids 96–7
Lung necrosis 123
Lupus erythematosus 152, 278
Lupus vulgaris 36, 152, 253
Lutzomyia spp., *see* Sandflies
Lyme disease 278
Lymph node involvement in tuberculosis 129, 134–6
Lymphadenitis, tuberculous 135
Lymphadenopathy 279
　AIDS-related 147, 232
　chancroid 176
　leishmaniasis 26
　pulmonary tuberculosis 132
　rickettsial disease 194
　trypanosomal 42
Lymphatic damage, filarial 103
Lymphatic leukaemia 5
Lymphoedema, chronic 103, 104
Lymphogranuloma venereum 177–8
Lymphoma 27, 43, 136, 139

MacKay-Dick reaction 157
Macules, leprous 149, 150
Madurella mycetomatosis 249
Malabsorption 68, 70, 213
Malaria 11, 43, 170, 185, 186, 196, 224, 227, 239
　anaemia 8
　and bacterial infection 16
　cerebral 11, 13, 16, 277
　clinical features 8–10
　coma 8, 9
　control 18

diagnosis 10–11
epidemiology 3–4
fever 5, 8
hypoglycaemia 6
immunity 7, 9, 10
incubation 4
pathogenesis 5–8
and pregnancy 20
prophylaxis 18–21
renal failure 6, 7
sequestration 5–6
'severe and complicated' 5–7, 8, 9
splenomegaly 5, 8
transmission 3–5
treatment 12–18
vaccines 21
see also Plasmodium falciparum
Malignant spinal metastases 143
Malnutrition 259–62
  beri beri 263, 266
  goitre/cretinism 265
  kwashiorkor 259, 260, 261
  and malaria 7–8
  marasmus 259, 260, 261
  pellagra 263–4
  rickets 264
  see also Vitamin deficiency
Maloprim 19
Malathion 265
Mansonella spp. 102, 106
Marasmus 259, 260, 261
Mazzotti reaction 108
Measles 278
Measly food 90
Mebendazole 79, 86, 87, 98
Mefloquine 14, 19–20
Megacolon 51, 214
Megaoesophagus 50–1
Melarsoprol 44, 44–5
Melioidosis 186, 278
Meningism 158
Mengingitis 11, 277
  acute bacterial 167–68, 227
    haemophilus 165–7
    meningococcal 161–5, 196
    pneumococcal 167
  Cryptococcus 250
  cistericoid 92

  eosinophilic 275
  lymphocytic 156
  lymphomatous 235
  tuberculous 144–7, 234
Meningoencephalitis, *see*
    Trypanosomiasis, African
Menstrual disorders 142
Marburg fever *238*
Metagonimiasis 121
Metriphonate 112
Metronidazole 63, 64, 65, 70, 109
Microsporum canis 249
Miliary disease 43, 147, 185, 187
Mite-borne typhus 193, 198
Mitsuda reaction 151
Montenegro test 28, 33–4, 37
Mosquito 3, 4, 101, *102*; See also
    arbovirus; malaria
Moxibustion *152*
Murine typhus 192–3, 195, 198
Murray valley virus 224, 228
Myalgia 86, 156
Mycetoma 109, 249
Mycobacterium spp. 134, 138; *see also*
    Leprosy; tuberculosis
Myelofibrosis 27
Myiasis 253, 255

Nalidixic acid 215
Nasopharyngeal infection 161, 162, 166
Necator americanus, see Hookworms
Necrosis
  arterial wall 194
  enteritis 212, 212–13
  snake venom 267, 268, 269
Neisseria gonorrhoeae 180
Neisseria meningitidis 161–2
Nematode parasites *102*
Neomycin 291
Nephrotic syndrome 5
Neurofibromatosis *152*
Neuropathy
  leprous 150, 151
  peripheral *152*
Neurosyphilis 43
Niacin 265–6
Niclosamide 94

Nicotinic acid 263–4
Nifurtimox 52
Niridazole 109
Nystatin pessaries 182

O'nyong'nyong 224, 226
Obstruction, abdominal 139
Oedema 259
    periorbital 86
Onchocerca volvulus 102, 106, 106–7
Onchocerciasis 106–8, *152*
Onchomycosis 249
Ophthalmia neonatorum 183–4
Opisthorciasis 116–17
Oral rehydration (ORT) 163, 206, 207, 211, 215, 217, 261, 292
Organophosphate poisoning 174, 244, 265–6
Oriental sore 32–3, 35
    see also Leishmaniasis, cutaneous
Oropouche fever 224, 226
ORT, see Oral rehydration
Osteomalacia 264

Palsy 145, 150
Pancreatitis 78, 115
Pantothenic acid deficiency 266
Pancytopenia 26
Papilloedema 144
Paracoccidiodes brasiliensis 250
Paragonimiasis 122–5, 186
Paralysis
    diphtheria toxin 253
    organophosphate 265
    rabies 243
    snake bite 267, 268
Paraplegia, lathyritic 266
Parasympathetic denervation 51
Parathion 265
Paratyphoid infection 112
Pein bois *35*
Pelvic inflammatory disease 182–3
Penicillin 157, 163, 164–5, 167, 177, 181, 253
Pentamidine 44
Pentostam 28
Pericardial constriction 138
Pericardial friction rub 137

Pericardial tuberculosis 136–38
Pericarditis 136–7, 164
Peritonitis, tuberculous 139
Petechiae of meningococcaemia 162
Phenothiazine poisoning 174
Phenothiazines *238*
Phlebotomus spp.; see Sandflies
Photophobia, of rickettsial disease 194
Phytate ingestion, and rickets 264
Pig, infection from 91, 119, 120
Pig bel 212
Pituitary ischaemia 268
Pityriasis versicolor 249
PKDL (post kala-azar dermal leishmaniasis) 26–7, 28, *35, 154*
Plague 187, 188, 188–9, 279
Plasmodia spp. 3–4
    see also Malaria
Plasmodia falciparum
    malaria 5–7
    sequestration 5–6
    drug resistance 12–13, 14–15
    infection 11–12
Pleural reaction 130
Pleural rub 59–60
Pneumococcal meningitis 167
Pneumocystis carinii 250–1
Pneumonia *238*
    bacteraemic, and pneumoccocal meningitis 167
    mycoplasmic 200
    pneumonic plague 188
    pneumonitis 278–9
    podoconiosis 104
    poisoning 11
        organophosphate 174, 244, 265–6
        phenothiazine 174
        Spanish toxic oil 86
        strychnine 174
Poliomyelitis 285–6
Polymorphism 8
Pork, parasites in 85
Post kala-azar dermal leishmaniasis, see PKDL
Potassium 207, 210
Potts disease 145

Praziquantel 94, 112, 116, 117, 118, 119, 120, 121, 122
Prednisolone 86, 138
Pregnancy
  ectopic 183
  and malaria 8, 20
  and mebendazole 79
  use of tetracycline 64
Primaquine 12, 13
Proguanil 12, 19
Pruritis 84
Pseudomonas pseudomallei 186
Pseudopolyposis of the colon 113
Psittacosis 200
Psoas abscess 143
Psoriasis 152
Pulmonary cavitation 131
Pulmonary collapse 130
Pulmonary eosinophilia 273, 279
Pulmonary hypertension 113
Pulmonary oedema, malarial 15
Pulmonary paragonimiasis 122–3
Pulmonary tuberculosis 130–4, 147
Pyopneumothorax 131
Pyrantel pamoate (Combantrin) 79, 82
Pyrazinamide 133, 146
Pyrexia, *see* Fever
Pyridoxine deficiency 266
Pyrimethamine 12

Q fever 170, 185, 199–200, *238*, 279
Quinine 14, 15, 16, 17, 18
Quinolone antibiotics 291

Rabies 227, 243–5, 289
Rash
  arbovirus 278
  dengue fever 225
  louse-borne typhus 194–5
  Q fever 199
  relapsing fever 158
  scrub typhus 195
  typhoid 169
Rat, as typhus reservoir 192
Rectal prolapse 87
Rectal stricture 178
Reduviid bug 47, 48–9

Rehydration, *see* Oral rehydration
Relapsing fever 11, 196, 224, 278
  louse-born 158–9
  tick-borne 160
Relapsing malaria 4
Renal failure
  malarial 6, 7, 15
  snake bite 268
Renal hydatids 97
Renal tuberculosis 141–2
Resistance, *see* Drug resistance
Respiratory tract, AIDS infection 233
Retinitis 234
Retinol 262
Reversal reaction 150–1, 152
Rheumatic fever 279
Ribavarin 241
Rickets 264
Rickettsialpox 194, 196
Rickettsioses 163
  clinical features 194
  control 198
  diagnosis 196–7
  ehrlichiosis *192*, 200–1
  Q fever *194*, 201–2
  spotted fever *192*, 194–5, 196, 278
  treatment 199–200
  typhus 191–3, 194–5
Rifampicin 131, 133, 136, 138, 141, 146, 151, 164, 185, *239*
Rift Valley fever 224, 229
Rodents 32, 157, 192
Romana's sign 50
Ross River fever 224, 226
Rubella 278

Salmonella (para)typhi 113, 169
Salmonellosis 61, 209–10, 278
  and AIDS 232
Salt intake 293
Sandflies
  control 29
  leishmaniasis 31, 32
  phlebotomine 23, 24–5
Sarcoidosis 36, 136, *152*
Scabies 180, 255, 274
Scalp fungal infection 249
Scarification *152*

Schistosomiasis 61, 111–14, 209, 210, 273
Scrofula, *see* Lymph-node tuberculosis
Scrub typhus 193, 195, 198, 279
Septicaemia 186, 188
Sequestration 5–6
Serological tests 62–3, 105
Sexually transmitted diseases (STD) 290–1
  chancroid 176
  gonorrhoea 180–1
  granuloma inguinale 179
  hepatitis B/D 239, 240, 241
  herpes 178–9
  lymphogranuloma venereum 177–78
  ophthalmia neonatorum 183–4
  pelvic inflammatory disease 182–3
  scabies 181
  syphilis 36, 177
  ulcer 175–80
  urethral discharge 180–1
  vaginal discharge 181–2
Sheehan's syndrome 268
Sheep liver fluke 117–18
Shigellosis 187, 213–15
Shock, in dengue 225
Sickle-cell disease 210, 253
Similum spp. (black fly) 107
Skin, *see* Dermatitis; Rash; Ulcer
Skin eruptions, hookworm induced 82–3
Sleeping sickness, *see* trypanosomiasis, African
Slim disease 74, 232, 261; *see also* AIDS; cryptosporidiosis
Small intestine
  inflammation 120
  parasitized 96
  strongyloidiasis 83
  tapeworms 89, 91
  Trichinella 85
Snails 110, 113–14, 275
  and liver flukes 115, 117–18, 119, 120, 121, 122
Snake bite 267–69
Spanish toxic oil poisoning 86
Spectinomycin 183

Spinal paragonimiasis 124
Spinal tuberculosis 142–4, 266
Spleen, granulomas in 185
Splenectomy, in leishmaniasis 28–9
Splenomegaly 27, 113
  brucellosis 185
  malarial 5, 8
  trypanosomal 50
  typhoid 169
Sporotrichosis 36, 250
Spotted fever 192, 193–4, 196, 278
Sprue 218–19
St Louis virus 224, 228
Steatorrhoea 84
Streptomycin 146
Stricture 178
Strongyloides stercoralis 83–4
Strongyloidiasis 83–5, 86, 273
  and Loeffler's pneumonia 78
Streptococcus pneumoniae 161, 167
Strychnine poisoning 174
Sulphonamides 12, 238
  resistance to 163, 164
Superior mesenteric vein, flukes in 111, 112
Suramin 44, 108
Swimmer's itch 112, 113
Syphilis 36, 177

T cell leukaemia 235
Tachycardi 137, 162
Taenia and Loeffler's pneumonia 78
Taenia saginata 89–91
Taenia solium 91–5
Tapeworms 89
  Echinococcus granulosus 95–8
  Echinocuccus multilocularis 98–9
  Taenia saginata 89–91
  Taenia solium 91–5
Tetanus 109, 173–4, 269
Tetracycline 159, 177, 181, 183, 185–6, 197, 198, 200, 201, 208, 219
Tetraplegia 145
Thiabendazole 38, 85, 88, 249
Thiacetazone 148
Thiamine, see vitamin B_1
Thiacetazone 133
Thiocyanate toxicity 266

Thrombocytopenia 201
Thrombotic occlusion 194
Tick typhus *192*, 194
Tick-borne infection
  encephalitis 228
  ehrlichiosis 200–1
  spotted fever 193–4, 196, 198
  relapsing fever 159
Tinea capitis 249
Tinidazole 63, 70
Toxocara spp. 88
Toxocariasis 86, 273
Toxoplasmosis 188, 279
TPE, *see* Tropical pulmonary eosinophilia
Transfusions 17
Trematodes, *see* Schistosomiasis: Fluke
Treponema pallidum 177
Trichinella and Loeffler's pneumonia 78
Trichinella spiralis 85
Trichinosis 85–7, 273
Trichomonas 182
Trichuriasis 87–8
Trichuris trichiura 78, 79, 87
Trismus 173
Tropical pulmonary eosinophilia (TPE) 103
Tropical spastic paraparesis (TSP) 235
Tropical sprue 218–19
Tropical ulcer 253
Trypanosoma brucei 39–40
  see also Trypansomiasis, African
Trypanosoma cruzi 47–8
  see also Trypanosomiasis, American
Trypanosomiasis 277, 278, 279
  African 39–46
    clinical features 42–4
    control 45–6
    diagnosis 43–4
    epidemiology 39–42
    reservoir 41–2
    treatment 44–5, 44–5
    vector 40–1, 45–6
  American 47–53*
    clinical features 49–52
    control 52–3
    diagnosis 51–2

epidemiology 47–9
reservoir 49
treatment 51
vector 47, 48–9
Tsetse fly 39, 40–1
Tuberculin test 131
Tuberculoid leprosy 150
Tuberculosis 129–30, 278, 279
  abdominal 138–41
  and AIDS 147–48, 233
  cerebral 43
  differential diagnosis 36, 43, 124, 185, 186, 187, 266
  genitourinary 141–2
  laryngitis 132
  lymph node 134–6
  meningitis (TBM) 145–7, 234
  miliary 43, 185, 187
  nutritional deficiency disease in 261
  pericardial 136–38
  peritonitis 139
  primary infection 130–1
  pulmonary 130–4, 147
  spinal 142–4, 266
Tuberculostearic acid 146
Tularaemia 187, 188, 200
Typhoid 11, 169–71, 185, 188, 196, 200, *238*, 277, 278, 279, 280
Typhus 11, 170, 188, 191–3, 277, 278, 279, 280
  mite-borne 193, 198

Ulcer
  amoebiasis 60
  amoebic dysentery 56–7
  chancroid 178
  granuloma inguinale 179
  herpes 180
  leishmaniasis 32–3, 34–6
  leprosy 150, 151
  lower leg 109
  scrub typhus 195
  skin 253
  syphilis 177
  tropical 253
Ultraviolet light 264
Upgrading reaction 150–1, 152

Ureteric colic 142
Uretheral discharge (male) 180–1
Urinary bladder vein, flukes in 112, 112–13
Urticaria 84

Vaccine
  arbovirus encephalitis 228
  BCG 134, 289
  Biken 288
  cholera 286–7
  Clostridium perfringens 213
  haemophilus meningitis 166–7
  hepatitis 237, 241, 287–88
  Japanese encaphalitis 288
  leishmaniasis 38
  malaria 21
  meningococcal meningitis 165, 289
  plague 188
  polio 285–6
  rabies 244, 289
  tetanus 174, 290
  typhoid 171, 286
  yellow fever 224–5, 289–90
Vaginal discharge 181–2
Vaginitis 181–2
Vasculitis 194
Venous pressure, high 137
Vermox 79

Vertebral body destruction 143
Vibrio chloera 205
Vibrio parahaemolyticus 209
Viper bite 267, 268
Viral gastroenteritis 219
Visceral dilatation 50, 51
Visceral larva migrans 88
Vision, and vitamin A 262
Vitamin deficiency
  A 259, 260, 262–3
  B_1 186, 263, 266
  B_{12} 70
  D 266–7
Vitiligo *152*
Volvulus 78

Weil-Felix test 197
Wernicke's encephalopathy 263
West Nile fever 224, 226
Widal test 170
Winterbottom's sign 42
Wuchereria bancrofti, see Filariasis

Yaws *152*, 253
Yellow fever 223–5, 228, *238*, 278
Yersinia enterocolitica 217
Yersinia pseudotuberculosis 188
Yersiniosis 187, 278
Yomesan 94